KETO DIET COOKBOOK FOR WOMAN AFTER 50

The complete Ketogenic Diet Guide for Seniors with 200+ Simple and Delicious Recipes; Reset your Metabolism and Stay Healthy with 28 Days Keto Meal Plan

Ashley Jones

© **Copyright 2020 by Ashley Jones - All rights reserved.**

The content contained within this book may not be reproduced, duplicated or transmitted without direct written permission from the author or the publisher.

Under no circumstances will any blame or legal responsibility be held against the publisher, or author, for any damages, reparation, or monetary loss due to the information contained within this book. Either directly or indirectly.

Legal Notice:

This book is copyright protected. This book is only for personal use. You cannot amend, distribute, sell, use, quote or paraphrase any part, or the content within this book, without the consent of the author or publisher.

Disclaimer Notice:

Please note the information contained within this document is for educational and entertainment purposes only. All effort has been executed to present accurate, up to date, and reliable, complete information. No warranties of any kind are declared or implied. Readers acknowledge that the author is not engaging in the rendering of legal, financial, medical or professional advice. The content within this book has been derived from various sources. Please consult a licensed professional before attempting any techniques outlined in this book.

By reading this document, the reader agrees that under no circumstances is the author responsible for any losses, direct or indirect, which are incurred as a result of the use of information contained within this document, including, but not limited to, — errors, omissions, or inaccuracies.

Introduction

Is Keto Right for You?

Growing old is part of life, but one can retain an active and healthy lifestyle long into your later years.

The aging process affects the body in many ways. As we age, our bodies undergo a variety of changes. Our hair begins to gray; our skin loses its elasticity, and wrinkles develop. Muscle loss, thinning skin, and reduced stomach acids are all a part of the aging process. Most of the changes will make you more susceptible to weight gain while also causing nutrient deficiencies. For example, reduced acids in your stomach can affect how nutrients are being absorbed, such as Iron, Vitamin b12, calcium, and magnesium.

Compounding these issues is that as we age, our bodies require less fuel, and we need to decrease the number of calories we eat in a day. This makes it challenging to make sure we get the nutrients needed while eating fewer calories. It's a bit of a nutritional dilemma.

Lucky for us, there are several steps you can do to prevent deficiencies and other age-related changes. As an example, consuming food that is rich in nutrients and ingesting the right supplements can aid in keeping you healthy as you age. Following a Keto-diet is one great way of staying healthy as you continue to age.

The choices we make regarding our food on a day to day basis and over our lifetime will always matter more than ever. It may occur to you that since the Keto diet does not allow processed foods and carbohydrates that it is a highly restrictive diet. The Keto diet is not restrictive, as far as diet plans go. As long as you stay to the allowed food groups, you will be given free rein to decide what you want to eat. You will not be experience boredom since choices of food because there are so many choices available. Here in this book, we will be listing down all the foods you can and can't eat.

Everyone knows that watching what you eat and staying active is vital to a healthy lifestyle. However, as we age, things just aren't that simple. Our nutritional needs evolve. Many women find themselves suffering from physical disorders that can make it difficult to swallow, digest foods properly, or find themselves with a significantly reduced appetite.

Your diet is linked to your immune function; it influences mental health and is critical in maintaining healthy bones and sharp eyes. That means women over 50 should make eating a healthy diet suited to their specific needs the highest priority.

Developing and implementing a Keto-friendly diet plan will help to ensure that you are eating nutrient-rich foods while eliminating calorie-dense foods that hold no nutritional value.

Because of its focus on eating nutrient-dense foods, the Keto-diet is perfect for women over 50. With some tweaking and a few minor adjustments to reduce caloric intake and different nutritional needs, this diet can be tailored to meet everyone's individual needs.

Read this guide for more on how to approach the Keto diet after 50.

CONTENTS

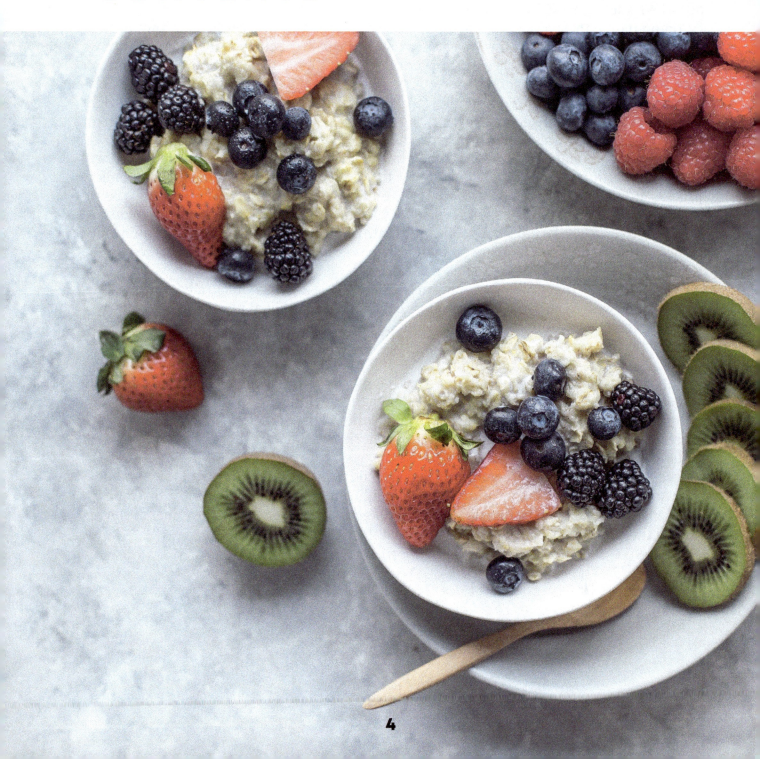

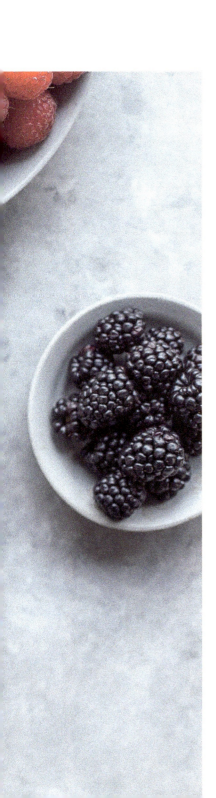

8	BODY CHANGES AFTER 50 AND WHY IT'S BEEN SO HARD FOR YOU TO LOSE
11	WHY SHOULD YOU CHOOSE KETO DIET EVEN IF YOU'RE
14	BENEFITS OF KETO DIET
17	WHAT ARE MACROS, CALORIES AND HOW TO TRACK THEM
21	HOW TO CUSTOMIZE YOUR KETO DIET
26	COMMON MISTAKES AND HOW TO AVOID THEM
29	FOODS TO EAT AND FOODS TO AVOID
34	28 DAY MEAL PLAN
36	SHOPPING LIST

40 RECIPES

40	BREAKFAST
68	APPETIZERS AND SIDES
92	SEAFOOD
120	POULTRY
145	MEAT
174	VEGETABLES
203	SOUPS AND STEWS
230	SNACKS
246	DESSERTS
276	DRINKS

i CONCLUSION

1

BODY CHANGES AFTER 50

For women, the most significant changes happen at 50. All of these changes are natural occurrences that every woman experience as a result of their aging process.

These changes don't only bring bad symptoms with them, but they also have a severe adverse effect on your hormones, too.

Insulin

Insulin resistance which can lead to a spike in blood sugar is caused by low estrogen levels. The hormone, insulin is made by the pancreas that is responsible in regulating the levels of glucose in the blood. When one has resistance to insulin, the cells does not allow glucose to enter which leaves sugar in the blood flowing free in your bloodstream. This will lead to health issues such as weight gain and diabetes.

Ghrelin

During aging, many women will have higher levels of ghrelin also known as hunger hormone, known for stimulating the fat and promoting the storage of fat in the body.

The ghrelin levels are increased. You feel hungry and trigger the reward center of the brain. Your appetite for food will be higher. The process of digestion gets fast and will let calories to be absorbed at a higher rate. The ghrelin in your stomach gets released even speedier.

Due to higher levels of ghrelin, women in the age of 50 struggles with experience increased abdominal fat and weight gain.

This can also cause hot flashes, mood swings, insomnia, fatigue and many more. Keto diet may help in managing these symptoms and regain the balance in your hormones.

Women over 50 – and those that have already been affected by menopause – besides the menopausal symptoms, in general, share three other health issues in common: low stomach acid, low thyroid function, and a sluggish gallbladder.

Low Stomach Acid

As we grow older, our stomach slows down the production of necessary acid, so most women se do not have the adequate levels of acid for their stomachs to be functioning normally. This is an important issue that needs to be addressed. However, if thinking about starting a Ketogenic diet, low stomach acid should be specially regulated as it plays an essential role in the digestion of protein and eliminating harmful microbes.

Thankfully, regulating stomach acid isn't that tricky. Depending on the severity of your condition, you can restore your gut balance without any special supplements. Doctors say that simply squeezing lemon juice or sprinkling apple cider vinegar over your meat and veggies will help you pre-metabolize the food you consume, which will aid digestion.

To boost the quality of your digestive juices, make sure to consume more fermented foods such as sauerkraut and kimchi, fermented drinks such as coconut kefir, and up the ginger intake.

Another trick that can help you improve stomach acid is to be mindful of consuming drinks during meals. Keep in mind that drinking plenty of water with meals only dilutes your digestive juices, making sure to leave the hydration outside the meals.

Also, make sure to time your protein consumption. It is best to eat protein-rich foods at the beginning of the meal for better stomach acid support.

If your condition is more severe and these simple strategies don't do you much good, then you should probably take supplements half-way through mealtimes.

Low Thyroid Function

Thyroid dysfunctions are not a strange occurrence for women and are especially common for older women. Women over 50 often struggle with hypothyroidism (low function) and experience lower vitality, unstable mood, decreased energy and increased weight.

Choosing the Keto lifestyle should take care of the problem if your thyroid hormones are not significantly imbalanced. Burning fat for energy and depriving your body of glucose should make women more flexible metabolically and stabilizes their blood sugar, which should, in turn, support a balanced production of the thyroid hormones.

But if you are suffering from hypothyroidism, you shouldn't put all your money on this Keto benefit. If your thyroid hormones are not balanced, then you should also address this issue by making sure to consume an adequate number of calories. If your body doesn't receive enough calories, it may go to a conservation state and experience a drop in the T3 thyroid hormone.

Those of you who are seriously struggling with hypothyroidism will benefit the most from a Ketogenic diet combined with carb cycling to increase the calorie intake.

Sluggish Gallbladder

Having a sluggish gallbladder may not seem like an incredibly severe issue, but it can indeed lead to many health-concerning issues. And besides, if you are willing to give the Keto diet a try, restoring gallbladder health and bile production is a definite must. Why? Because the gallbladder is known to be the reservoir for bile, and bile being a digestive juice that helps the fat emulsion and the creation of fatty acids, you can easily connect the dots and see why it is so important when you are utilizing ketones for energy.

There are many ways in which you can improve bile production and restore your gallbladder health. Supporting the stomach acid, eating smaller meals, and staying hydrated can all do wonders for your gallbladder.

The Rate of Metabolism Becomes Slow

When there is a decrease in muscle mass, the body's metabolic rate tends to slow down. Metabolism is a very complicated process that helps in the conversion of calories into useful energy. Having less muscle and more fat will reduce the calorie-burning process. Also, many people tend to get less active with growing age. It can also slow down the metabolism. Age is not the primary thing that can determine the metabolic rate. The sex and size of the body also play essential roles. Certain types of health conditions, like hypothyroidism, can also affect the rate of metabolism.

Not Enough Sleep

Not getting enough sleep and sleep disturbances are very common as you cross the mark of 50. For women, menopause can lead to sleep disruptions because of hot flashes or even arthritis. When you do not get enough sleep, it readily affects the overall production of the growth hormone. Growth hormone is essential for muscle and bone mass.

2

WHY SHOULD YOU CHOOSE KETO DIET EVEN IF YOU'RE 50+?

When you reach the age of 50, you will notice many changes in your body. Among the most common symptoms are a loss of muscle, the need for less sleep, and more refined skin. You don't have to worry about this. Still, you have to pay much more attention than usual to your lifestyle. It is essential to keep fit, get exercise, and have a healthy and correct diet under all macros.

From this perspective, the ketogenic diet offers enormous advantages. You can apply it even if you have health problems. Of course, a visit to a nutritionist can help you personalize your diet even more effectively. But this is "something more," the information in this book is more than enough. You just need to study it and apply it diligently.

As said, the functions of our body change according to age. The thing that changes most is our metabolism; it is physiological that it slows down with age. This change is due both to aging but also to our lifestyle. Current metabolism is a consequence of our lifestyle in recent years.

A healthy lifestyle, with frequent, low-abundance meals, with moderate alcohol consumption, will have a faster metabolism than a lifestyle consisting of large meals eaten once a day, alcohol, and insomnia.

The ketogenic diet can help you from this point of view, eliminating carbohydrates and promoting the elimination of fats from our body. Another advantage is its flexibility; in fact, you can play with macros and adapt them to your needs, lifestyle, and progress made, of course.

Start gradually; your body has adapted for years to an unhealthy lifestyle, so do not overdo it overnight. Take your time and slowly reach your goals. There is no need to run; this is a marathon, not 100 meters.

At first, you may feel tired, tired, without energy. Don't worry; it's a normal thing; it's your body adapting to the new food style. You're taking away its primary source of energy, carbohydrates; logically, it has to adapt. It must change the primary energy source, it must switch to using fats, but this takes time, two or three days are necessary. The drop-in sugars could decrease your pressure for a couple of days, avoid exercise, and there will be no problems. The resulting benefits will be enormous.

Women go through so much in life, don't we? From growing up, discovering the joys of life, pursuing a promising career, becoming a mother, there is so much that changes within such a short period.

While that is a part of life, what anyone would genuinely try and avoid would be putting on excessive weight that we carry around like unneeded luggage. It is embarrassing, it is distracting, and it is causing quite a few internal issues.

If you thought the biggest hurdle you will face when you hit 50 is a big belly, think again. This isn't the only problem we face. While some would say that having a generous belly is the biggest problem, I firmly believe that there are more severe issues to worry about than that. When it comes to women, well, things aren't looking good.

Our bodies, since birth, continuously change. Most of these changes do not harm us and are only natural. However, once we enter into our 50s, things are a lot different. Now, any changes within our body will directly affect how we perform, operate, and work. If we were to keep these changes unchecked and pay no close attention, things would take a worse turn.

Most of these issues will remain the same for men; however, due to the chemistry of our bodies and differences, both internal and external, both would face a variety of issues exclusive to their gender.

There are a few ways we can avoid these issues. Some of these ways require you to go back in time and start working out from a very young age, control your diet, and change your habits. That is the stuff of science fiction and hence is out of the equation.

Other ways would include visiting a doctor and getting pills and energy boosters to feel better while taking more pills to fight diabetes, high blood pressure, and other health issues. This way is not just hectic but far too complicated as well.

For a very long time, the only other way was to avoid worrying too much and hope that life would fix issues itself, and that never ended well for many. People have then left with worry and a gap that nothing was able to fill. In comes the ketogenic diet.

Call it a need of the hour, a savior in disguise, or anything you like. The fact remains that this is proving to be a popular option that is not only delivering results but is also helping millions to maintain a healthy lifestyle and reverse some of the damage their bodies have suffered.

Numerous studies have supported the idea that Keto diets are far more effective for older men and women than the younger folks. With so much to look forward to and so little to sacrifice, it does make sense to state that Keto is essentially becoming your permanent way of life once you hit 50, but why is that? Why do I and so many others proclaim Keto as an essential lifestyle choice for women above 50? The answer to this involves some explanation, but I will do my best to do just that!

As a woman, you have likely experienced significant differences in how you must diet compared to how men can diet. Women tend to have a more challenging time losing weight because of their different hormones and how their bodies break down fats. Another factor to consider is your age group. As the body ages, it is essential to be more attentive with the way that you care for yourself. Aging bodies start to experience problems more quickly, which can be avoided with the proper diet and exercise plan. Keto works well for women of all ages, and this is because of how it communicates with the body. No matter how fit you are right now or how much weight you need or want to lose, Keto will change the way that your body metabolizes, giving you a very personalized experience.

When starting your Keto diet, you should not be thinking about extremes because that isn't what Keto should be about. You should be able to place your body into ketosis without feeling terrible in the process. One of the essential guidelines to follow while starting your Keto journey is to listen to your body regularly. If you ever feel that you are starving or thoroughly disappointed, you will likely have to modify the way you are eating because it isn't reaching ketosis properly. It is not an overnight journey, so you need to remember to be patient with yourself and your body. Adapting to a Keto diet takes a bit of transition time and a lot of awareness.

The health benefits of the Keto diet are not different for men or women, but the speed at which they are reached does differ. As mentioned, women's bodies are a lot different when it comes to how they can burn fats and lose weight. For example, by design, women have at least 10% more body fat than men. No matter how fit you are, this is just an aspect of being a woman you must consider. Don't be hard on yourself if you notice that it seems like men can lose weight easier — that's because they can! What women have in additional body fat, men typically have the same in muscle mass. This is why men tend to see faster external results. That added muscle mass means that their metabolism rates are higher. That increased metabolism means that fat and energy get burned faster. When you are on Keto, though, the internal change is happening right away.

Your metabolism is unique, but it will also be slower than a man's by nature. Since muscle can burn more calories than fat, the weight just seems to fall off men, giving them the ability to reach the opportunity for muscle growth quickly. This should not be something that holds you back from starting your Keto journey. As long as you keep these realistic bodily factors in mind, you won't be left wondering why it takes you a little longer to start losing weight. This point will come for you, but it will take a bit more of a process you must be committed to following through with.

When the body begins to run on fats successfully, you have an automatic fuel reserve waiting to be burned. It will take some time for your body to do this. However, when it does, you will eat fewer calories and still feel full because your body knows to take energy from the fat you already have. This will become automatic. However, it is a process that requires some patience, but being aware of what is going on with your body can help you stay motivated while on Keto.

Because a Keto diet reduces the amount of sugar you are consuming, it naturally lowers insulin in your bloodstream. This can have tremendous effects on any existing PCOS and fertility issues and menopausal symptoms and conditions like pre-diabetes and Type 2 diabetes. Once your body adjusts to a Keto diet, you are overcoming the naturally in place that can prevent you from losing weight and getting healthy. Even if you placed your body on a strict diet, if it isn't getting rid of sugars properly, you likely aren't going to see the same results you will when you try Keto. This is a big reason why Keto can be so beneficial for women.

For women over 50, there are guidelines to follow when you start your Keto diet. As long as you follow the method correctly and listen to what your body truly needs, you should have no more problems than men do while following the plan. What you will have are more obstacles to overcome, but you can do it. Remember that plenty of women successfully follow a Keto diet and see great results. Use these women as inspiration for how you anticipate your journey to go. When it seems impossible, remember what you have working against you and what you have working for you. Your body is designed to go into ketogenesis more than designed to store fat by overeating carbs. Use this as a motivation to keep pushing you ahead. Keto is a valid option for you, and the results will prove this, especially if you are over the age of 50.

3

BENEFITS OF KETO DIET

The Keto diet has become so popular in recent years because of the success people have noticed. Not only have they lost weight, but scientific studies show that the Keto diet can help you improve your health in many others. As when starting any new diet or exercise routine, there may seem to be some disadvantages, so we will go over those for the Keto diet. But most people agree that the benefits outweigh the change period!

Benefits/ Advantages

Losing weight: for most people, this is the foremost benefit of switching to Keto! Their previous diet method may have stalled for them, or they were noticing weight creeping back on. With Keto, studies have shown that people have been able to follow this diet and relay fewer hunger pangs and suppressed appetite while losing weight at the same time! You are minimizing your carbohydrate intake, which means more occasional blood sugar spikes. Often, those fluctuations in blood sugar levels make you feel hungrier and more prone to snacking in between meals. Instead, by guiding the body towards ketosis, you are eating a more fulfilling diet of fat and protein and harnessing energy from ketone molecules instead of glucose. Studies show that low-carb diets effectively reduce visceral fat (the fat you commonly see around the abdomen increases as you become obese). This reduces your risk of obesity and improves your health in the long run.

Reduce the Risk of Type 2 Diabetes: The problem with carbohydrates is how unstable they make blood sugar levels. This can be very dangerous for people who have diabetes or are pre-diabetic because of unbalanced blood sugar levels or family history. Keto is an excellent option because of the minimal intake of carbohydrates it requires. Instead, you are harnessing most of your calories from fat or protein, which will not cause blood sugar spikes and, ultimately, less pressured the pancreas to secrete insulin. Many studies have found that diabetes patients who followed the Keto diet lost more weight and eventually reduced their fasting glucose levels. This is monumental news for patients with unstable blood sugar levels or hopes to avoid or reduce their diabetes medication intake.

Improve cardiovascular risk symptoms to lower your chances of having heart disease: Most people assume that following Keto is so high in fat content has to increase your risk of coronary heart disease or heart attack. But the research proves otherwise! Research shows that switching to Keto can lower your blood pressure, increase your HDL good cholesterol, and reduce your triglyceride fatty acid levels. That's because the fat you are consuming on Keto is healthy and high-quality fats, so they reverse many unhealthy symptoms of heart disease. They boost your "good" HDL cholesterol numbers and decrease your "bad" LDL cholesterol numbers. It also reduces the level of triglyceride fatty acids in the bloodstream. A top-level of these can lead to stroke, heart attack, or premature death. And what are the top levels of fatty acids linked to?

High Consumption of Carbohydrates: With the Keto diet, you are drastically cutting your intake of carbohydrates to improve fatty acid levels and improve other risk factors. A 2018 study on the Keto diet found that it can improve 22 out of 26 risk factors for cardiovascular heart disease! These factors can be critical to some people, especially those who have a history of heart disease in their family.

Increases the Body's Energy Levels: Let's briefly compare the difference between the glucose molecules synthesized from a high carbohydrate intake versus ketones produced on the Keto diet. The liver makes ketones and use fat molecules you already stored. This makes them much more energy-rich and an endless source of fuel compared to glucose, a simple sugar molecule. These ketones can give you a burst of energy physically and mentally, allowing you to have greater focus, clarity, and attention to detail.

Decreases inflammation in the body: Inflammation on its own is a natural response by the body's immune system, but when it becomes uncontrollable, it can lead to an array of health problems, some severe and some minor. The health concerns include acne, autoimmune conditions, arthritis, psoriasis, irritable bowel syndrome, and even acne and eczema. Often, removing sugars and carbohydrates from your diet can help patients of these diseases avoid flare-ups - and the delightful news is Keto does just that! A 2008 research study found that Keto decreased a blood marker linked to high inflammation in the body by nearly 40%. This is glorious news for people who may suffer from inflammatory disease and want to change their diet to improve.

Increases your mental Functioning Level: As we elaborated earlier, the energy-rich ketones can boost the body's physical and mental levels of alertness. Research has shown that Keto is a much better energy source for the brain than simple sugar glucose molecules are. With nearly 75% of your diet coming from healthy fats, the brain's neural cells and mitochondria have a better source of energy to function at the highest level. Some studies have tested patients on the Keto diet and found they had higher cognitive functioning, better memory recall, and were less susceptible to memory loss. The Keto diet can even decrease the occurrence of migraines, which can be very detrimental to patients.

Decreases risk of diseases like Alzheimer's, Parkinson's, and epilepsy. They created the Keto diet in the 1920s to combat epilepsy in children. From there, research has found that Keto can improve your cognitive functioning level and protect brain cells from injury or damage. This is very good to reduce the risk of neurodegenerative disease, which begins in the brain because of neural cells mutating and functioning with damaged parts or lower than peak optimal functioning. Studies have found that the following Keto can improve the mental functioning of patients who suffer from diseases like Alzheimer's or Parkinson's. These neurodegenerative diseases sadly have no cure, but the Keto diet could improve symptoms as they progress. Researchers believe that it's because of cutting out carbs from your diet, which reduces the occurrence of blood sugar spikes that the body's neural cells have to keep adjusting to.

Keto can regulate hormones in women who have PCOS (polycystic ovary syndrome) and PMS (pre-menstrual syndrome). Women who have PCOS suffer from infertility, which can be very heartbreaking for young couples trying to start a family. For this condition, there is no known cure, but we believe it's related to many similar diabetic symptoms like obesity and a high level of insulin. This causes the body to produce more sex hormones, which can lead to infertility. The Keto diet paved its way as a popular way to regulate insulin and hormone levels and increase a woman's chances of getting pregnant.

Disadvantages

Your body will have a Changed period: It depends from person to person on the number of days that will be, but when you start any new diet or exercise routine, your body has to adjust to the new normal. With the Keto diet, you are drastically cutting your carbohydrates intake, so the body must adjust to that. You may feel slow, weak, exhausted, and like you are not thinking as quick or fast as you used to. It just means that your body is making adjustments to Keto, and once this change period is done, you will see the weight loss results you expected.

If you are an athlete, you may need more carbohydrates: If you still want to try Keto as an athlete, you must talk to your nutritionist or trainer to see how the diet can be tweaked for you. Most athletes require a greater intake of carbs than the Keto diet requires, which means they may have to up their intake to ensure they have the energy for their training sessions. High endurance sports (like rugby or soccer) and heavy weightlifting require more significant information on carbohydrates. If you're an athlete wanting to follow Keto and gain the health benefits, it's crucial you first talk to your trainer before changing your diet.

You have to count your daily macros carefully: For beginners, this can be tough, and even people already on Keto can become lazy about this. People are often used to eating what they want without worrying about just how many grams of protein or carbs it contains. With Keto, be meticulous about counting your intake to ensure you are maintaining the Keto breakdown (75% fat, 20% protein, ~5% carbs). The closer you stick to this, the better results you will see regarding weight loss and other health benefits. If your weight loss has stalled or you're not feeling as energetic as you hoped, it could be because your macros are off. Find a free calorie counting app that you look at the ingredients of everything you're eating and cooking.

4

WHAT ARE MACROS, CALORIES AND HOW TO TRACK THEM

Your macronutrients or **"macros"** stand for the amount of fat, protein, and carbohydrates in your foods. When you calculate your numbers, this refers to the number of grams you will consume in a given day. If you have no idea what I am talking about, this is perfect for you.

We will be discussing each of the three macronutrients, how to balance them, and how to calculate your macros for the ketogenic diet. All three nutrients will be vital if you are looking to get into and stay in ketosis while following a ketogenic diet.

What Are Macros?

Before we dive into specifics, you must understand what macros even are in the first place! Macros are the three main macronutrients humans need to survive. The three main macros include fat, protein, and carbohydrate. Within these three nutrients, we receive the micronutrients such as minerals and vitamins that we need to stay alive.

Depending on the diet plan you are looking at, macronutrients will have different ratios. Obviously, on the ketogenic diet, it will be high fat, moderate protein, and low carbohydrates. Finding the balance of these three macronutrients is essential because they contribute to your energy levels. When you come up with the sum of the calories you consumed for each group, this will give you your calorie intake for the day. This figure is essential for us who are looking to lose weight on the ketogenic diet. For now, let's take a more in-depth look into each macronutrient and why it is essential.

Fats

While society has been teaching us that fat is wrong, we need fat to survive. This fat you will be eating is vital for several reasons, mostly because it is about to become your primary energy source. On top of this reason, fats also help the body carry and absorb vitamins such as A, D, E, and K, which are needed for body functions. Other fats that are essential for your health are omega-3 and omega-6 fatty acids.

There are healthy and less healthy fats; you must understand the difference before beginning your ketogenic diet. Below, we will go over several types to know what to eat and what to avoid.

Saturated Fats

The first fat we will be discussing is saturated fat. This type of fat comes from the fatty part of an animal product. This is typically the fat found in dairy products, meat trimmings, lard, and butter. While overeating this fat can raise your LDL or bad cholesterol, it is acceptable in moderation on the ketogenic diet.

Monounsaturated Fatty Acids (MUFA)

These types of fats are generally healthier for you and are plant-based. Some more common sources of MUFAs are peanut butter, avocado, canola oil, and olive oil. These are excellent sources as they can reduce bad cholesterol, reduce the risk of cardiovascular disease.

Polyunsaturated Fatty Acids (PUFA)

If you are looking to get more omega-3 and omega-6 fatty acids in your diet, you will want to look for PUFAs. Some of the significant sources of this include flaxseed, tofu, sunflower seeds, and walnuts. PUFAs are essential to include in your diet as they can decrease your risk of cardiovascular disease and lower your LDL. On top of these benefits, a proper balance of PUFAs in your diet can help with immune functions, neural functions, and other biological functions within your body.

Trans Fats

This is the fact that you are going to want to avoid while following the ketogenic diet. Trans fats exist as a product of significant processing in foods. They are found in store-bought goodies and commercially fried foods. Unfortunately, this type of fat can make your cholesterol sky-high and increases your risk of cardiovascular disease. If you see any trans fats in your foods, drop them.

As far as how much fat you need to consume on your diet that will depend on your goals for your new diet. In general, if you are looking to lose weight, you need to eat less fat until you start losing weight. If you are looking to gain muscle, you're going to eat fat until you gain weight! We are all on different journeys. To figure out what your macros should be, I suggest using an online calculator.

Proteins

Next, we will take a more in-depth look into proteins. While fat will make up a mass majority of your diet, it will be essential to balance it with a moderate amount of protein. Moderation is key here; frequently, beginners go overboard with their protein sources and hinder their results on the ketogenic diet.

Look at protein as the building block for your body. All of your tissues, including nail, hair, skin, and muscles, will rely on the proper amount of protein in your diet. Protein is also in charge of creating hemoglobin, a molecule that carries oxygen and prevents swelling and bloating.

The amount of protein you must have in your diet will vary depending on your body composition, body weight, activity levels, and body composition goals. For general purposes, you can stick with the following ranges to help keep yourself in ketosis:

- Not Active: 0.8g of protein per lean body mass.
- Light Activity: 0.8-1.0g of protein per lean body mass.
- High Activity: 1.0-1.2g of protein per lean body mass.

Protein is essential to your diet for several reasons. First, it will grant you the ability to maintain your muscle mass. When you begin the ketogenic diet, you probably want to lose some fat, but you need to make sure that you are not bringing your muscle down with it. Be sure to eat protein and exercise to keep yourself healthy and fit.

Protein is also vital to your diet as it can increase that feeling that you are full and keep your cravings at bay. When you are satisfied with the amount you are eating, this will help you eat fewer calories and, in turn, aiding you in losing more weight without feeling like you are starving all of the time. Protein also helps with weight loss as it can burn more calories compared to eating fat or carbs. The metabolism to burn protein requires more energy than carb or fat metabolism.

Carbohydrates

Finally, we end with carbohydrates. Remember that up until this point, the glucose your body has been running off of comes from this favorite fuel source, carbs. What is essential to know about carbohydrates is that there are two main carbohydrates, including simple and complex.

The reason carbs are classified into these two different groups is due to their chemical structure. Simple carbs will include fruit juices, potatoes, cookies, rice, bread, pasta, and cakes, all of which you already know is a big no-no on the ketogenic diet. The issue with simple carbs is that they contain a high amount of carbs, minimal amounts of fiber, and cause that "crash" in the afternoon after spike your blood sugar.

Complex carbs, on the other hand, include your vegetables, fruits, oatmeal, beans, quinoa, and whole-grain products. While most of these are still a no-go on the ketogenic diet, they contain the fiber that will benefit your diet. Please remember to refer to the section above to remember the carb foods you can and cannot include on the ketogenic diet.

Now that you have learned a gist about macronutrients, it will be up to you to find your ratios. As mentioned earlier, I highly suggest using an online calculator to find your numbers. We all make different plans for our lives and look to get something different from your new diet.

For menopausal and post-menopausal women, the best starting place is the Classic Keto Plan, which involves 75% fat, 20% protein, and only 5% of carbs.

Now that you know what your percentage should look like, let's go through how you can actually calculate the number of grams of each of these macronutrients that you should consume on a daily basis.

Because, remember, the Ketogenic diet should not be a dietary plan designed equally for everyone. The macro percentage of the classic Keto diet may be the same, but it should be calculated with your daily calorie intake in mind. Otherwise, how on earth can you manage to determine how much you should eat.

Once you find your ideal calorie amount, you can calculate your macros with three simple equations. But, before we do that, it is essential for you to know that the calories consumed from fat are not the same as the calories that you consume through carbs and protein:

- 1 gram of FAT = 9 calories
- 1 gram of CARBS = 4 calories
- 1 gram of PROTEIN = 4 calories

FAT

Here is how you can calculate how many grams of fat you should eat:

Daily Calories X Fat Percentage = Fat Calories / 9

So, let's assume that you've chosen to consume 2,000 calories a day. With that in mind, we can calculate the grams of fat this way:

2,000 x 0.75 (the percentage of fat on a classic Keto diet) = 1500 / 9 = 166

So, on a 2,000-calorie diet, you should consume 166 grams of fat per day.

On a 1,800-calorie diet, this would be 150 grams, on a 1,600-calorie diet, you should consume 133 grams of fat, and so on.

PROTEIN

Protein can be calculated the same way, only this time, we divide by 4 and we input the protein percentage:

Daily Calories X Protein Percentage = Protein Calories / 4

If you've chosen to consume 2,000 calories a day, you can calculate the protein this way:

2,000 x 0.2 = 400 / 4 = 100

On a 2,000-calorie diet, you should consume 100 grams of protein per day.

If you want your calorie intake to be 1,800, then you should consume 90 grams of protein, for a calorie intake of 1,600 you should consume 80 grams of protein, and so on.

CARBOHYDRATES

The formula for calculating the carbs is the same as for protein, with the percentage of carbs being the only difference:

Daily Calories X Carb Percentage = Carbohydrate Calories / 4

For 2,000 calories, the carbs should be calculated this way:

2,000 x 0.05 = 100 / 4 = 25

If you want to consume 2,000 calories a day, then you should limit your carb intake to 25 grams of NET carbs per day.

On a 1,800-calorie diet consume no more than 22.5 grams of NET carbs, on a 1,600-calorie diet limit the NET carb intake to 20 grams of NET carbs, and so on.

5

HOW TO CUSTOMIZE YOUR KETO DIET

There are many options when it comes to structuring your daily meals. The bottom line is that there is no one-size-fits-all approach for this, and it really comes down to your schedule, eating habits, and ultimately what allows you to feel most satisfied while maintaining a balanced Keto macro intake.

Once you're past the first week and getting the hang of consuming fewer carbohydrates, adequate-protein, and more healthy fats, you will most likely start to feel more satiated and notice that you can go for more extended periods without eating or snacking while still maintaining high energy, mood, and focus levels.

Make it a lifestyle. Figure out the meal timing that fits your schedule, keep you feeling satisfied throughout the day, and allows you to enjoy your meals without triggering more stressors.

The switch from a sugar burner to a fat burner can take some time. Most of us have been running on carbohydrates and sugar our entire lives, and our bodies have no idea what it feels like to be in "fat-burning mode" indeed.

There are a few different phases that our bodies go through during the adjustment period to becoming Keto-adapted. Making sure you take the appropriate steps during each of these phases is crucial for long-term success. During this challenge, you will transition through phase 1 and into phase 2. Phase 3 will come with time.

Phase 1: Getting into Ketosis

Achieving ketosis may take about 2-3 days. But the transition can be challenging if you are not taking advantage of the proper tools. Be sure always to follow the rules and guidelines.

1. Cut the carbs. The first step toward producing ketones is to decrease the consumption of carbs. Aim for 30 grams or less of total carbs per day and adjust accordingly.
2. Consumed enough healthy fats. Throw your fear of fat foods out the window and pump your body with the fuel it needs for energy—fat! This will make the transition phase more effective in burning fat

3. Moderate protein. Consuming too much protein, especially on its own, may spike insulin levels and make it harder to get into ketosis. Pair proteins with fats and be mindful of your intake.

4. Replenish electrolytes and water. When your intakes of carbs are decreased, your body will start flushing out more water and takes sodium and other electrolytes with it. This can lead to symptoms of "Keto flu," which is in more detail here.

5. Avoid a severe caloric deficit. Do not attempt to reduce your caloric intake during the first few days. Eat the same quantity of food you usually eat while changing the macro composition: fewer carbs, moderate protein, and more fat.

6. Take it easy with exercise. Reduce the volume and intensity of exercise for the first few days (and maybe even during the first few weeks) to reduce the added stressors and promote a favorable transition. Focus on lighter activities like yoga and leisurely swims or walks.

Phase 2: Transitioning To Fat-Burning Mode

In phase 2, your body will start to transition to effectively using fat and ketones for fuel. This will result in higher feelings of fullness throughout the day, stable blood sugar levels, fewer cravings, endless energy, better mood, laser-sharp focus, etc. This will start at the end of the first week and last for another six to eight weeks, depending on your adherence and prior metabolic health.

1. Continue to replenish electrolytes. Don't skimp on your electrolytes. It's essential to continue replenishing these minerals (primarily sodium, magnesium, and potassium) every day, especially surrounding physical activity.

2. Extend your fasting window. Now that your blood sugar is beginning to stabilize and you're starting to feel more satiated during the day, try to reduce snacking, extend your morning fast, and shut the kitchen down earlier at night.

3. Reduce caloric intake for fat loss. As you become efficient at using fat and ketones for fuel while feeling more satiated during the day, you should naturally decrease the amount of food you're consuming. This will allow you to start burning excess body fat. Use the guidelines (Macronutrient Ratios for Weight Loss) as a starting place and adjust accordingly.

4. Don't chase ketones. If you regularly test ketones, you may start to reduce your urine or blood levels. This is because your body and cells are starting to become more efficient at using fatty acids and ketones for fuel, which is a good thing! See here for more details on testing ketones.

Phase 3: Becoming Metabolically Flexible/Efficient

Once this is achieved, usually after four to six months or even up to a year, most people can effectively maintain a low-carbohydrate lifestyle while incorporating healthy carb sources and enjoying occasional indulgences.

1. Know that this is not a diet, rather a lifestyle. If you look at Keto as a diet, you will not succeed in the long term. If you go back to what you were doing before, you will end up exactly where you started.

2. Experiment with small increases in protein and carbs. After you've completely transitioned from a sugar burner to a fat-burner, you can start to play around with your protein and carb threshold.

Some people can bump up their carb and protein intake while remaining in ketosis.

3. Ease of going in and out of ketosis. Now that you're a thriving fat-burner, your body will give you a bit more leeway when it comes to indulging in some carbs every once in a while. But don't use this as an excuse to eat a whole carton of ice cream.

Side Effects during the Keto Diet and How to Overcome Them

The Keto diet is quite simple, just eat 75% fats, 20% protein, and 5% carbs. It is a general practice, most ketogenic beginners follow, and they maintain their body quite quickly. However, when you cross the age of 50, there are many challenges which you have to go through. Below is the list of those challenges, along with their solutions.

Keto-Flu

An abrupt shift of diet, from the regular intake of carbs to a limited amount, can cause Keto-flu, also known as carb withdrawal. It usually occurs after one to two days of withdrawal. Its symptoms include headache, muscle soreness, poor focus, sugar cravings, brain fog, irritability, insomnia, or weakness. The body will take some time for it to jump from burning carbohydrates to burning fats. Therefore, an abrupt transformation of diet sends your body into starvation mode, giving you those unpleasant symptoms.

Solution:
- Stay well, hydrated.
- Electrolytes Supplementation.
- Consume More Healthy Fats.
- Consume exogenous Ketone Supplement.

Muscle Cramps and Dehydration

Carbs need water for their storage, unlike fats. Hence, instead of being retained, a smaller amount of water is stored during the Keto diet, and the kidneys excrete more amount of sodium. Due to this, you can quickly get dehydrated while on the Keto diet, especially at the beginning. Due to this condition, low electrolyte concentration and dehydration, muscle cramping is inevitable.

Solution:
- Consult your doctor and complain to him/her about the problems you are facing.
- Add electrolytes supplements three major electrolytes, such as potassium, sodium, and magnesium.
- Ensure drinking a lot of water to remain hydrated.

Insomnia

Although there is not any research that has shown the effect of a Keto diet on sleep deprivation, there some people who have complained about a lack of quality sleep during the Keto diet. If this is the case with you, then once in a while, eating some high–quality carbs before bed can prove to be of enormous help.

Solution:
Before sleeping, take one teaspoon of raw honey. This will give your body adequate high-quality carbs during your sleep.

Brain Fog

When you eat fewer carbs, your body demands it; "I am hungry, and I want something to eat." When its wish isn't accommodated, it makes you fuzzy-headed. This is the brain's way of demanding more glucose. Because, up until now, that's the only fuel it has ever known.

Solution:

The best solution to remedy this condition is to ignore it and keep eating fat only. Ultimately, your brain will adapt to its new fuel, and your head will become more apparent than ever before.

Constipation

Consuming carbs lesser than 20g of per day means insufficient fibers, which ultimately results in constipation and irritable bowel syndrome. Constipation also occurs when you are not drinking enough water. The following are some remedies to aid you in your constipation.

Solution:

- Add leafy and good vegetables in your diet.
- Try cyclical Keto from time to time.
- Add enough natural salt such as Himalayan pink salt in your diet.
- Always remain hydrated and take electrolyte supplements.
- Do exercise regularly; it will also help you in relieving constipation problems.
- Try to take the recommended dosage of a good-quality digestive enzyme before or after every meal.
- Consume psyllium husk every morning. Mix one teaspoon in 1/2 cup of water and let it sit for 1 minute before drinking.

Diarrhea

Some people have diarrhea difficulties while on the Keto diet. Your body may react this way because of an increasing amount of fat intake, as it isn't yet able to produce and store enough bile to break down all the fat you're eating.

Solution:

Reduce the amount of fat you're eating by at least 10 percent.

Simultaneously, increase the number of fermented foods in your diets such as kombucha, water kefir, sauerkraut, kimchi, or your favorite fermented vegetable.

Add apple cider vinegar to your drinks and salad dressings.

Consider trying an ox bile supplement.

To cure diarrhea, lower your fat intake for seven days—or until you have adapted to the new changes. Then, gradually increase your fat intake back up to where it was.

Keto Rash

Keto rash, also called prurigo pigmentosa, is an itchy red rash that can develop on the neck, chest, back, and armpit areas; it is neither dangerous nor life-threatening. Although very rare, it sometimes occurs when people follow a strict ketogenic diet, usually 80 percent fat or higher. Other causative agents are hormonal imbalances, allergen exposure, and gut bacteria.

Solution:

Support your skin with adequate supplements and anti-inflammatory foods such as DHA, omega-3 supplements, or turmeric latte.

Keep yourself away from irritants like heat, sweat, or friction.

Reintroduce some carbs in your diet, though avoid consuming a lot of bread.

6

COMMON MISTAKES AND HOW TO AVOID THEM

Let's now introduce the concept of ketosis: Ketosis is a condition in which the body obtains energy by burning fat and producing so-called ketones. Typically, this situation occurs when blood glucose levels rise due to a decrease in insulin. Low ketosis levels are normal, but when ketones increase a lot in a short time, they can also have serious adverse effects.

That is, ketosis is the condition that we must achieve. It is our final result, the reason why we started the ketogenic diet. Knowing this new concept, let's see what the main errors in the ketogenic diet are.

Give up before completing ketosis

Nutritional ketosis is a mandatory step and brings more or less evident and more or less long aftermath. These vary based on how much carbohydrate has been abused previously and how much our liver is overloaded.

While the body is moving from burning sugar to burning fat, we have the sensation of feeling "poisoned" and "weighed down."

They are the toxins that are rising and, time a week or two, and it starts to bloom again.

Other symptoms related to the ketosis that is taking place are:

- Bad breath
- Slight nausea
- An initial hunger for sugars
- Tiredness
- Nervousness
- A slight sadness

These latter symptoms are linked to the impact that the elimination of sugars and carbohydrates has on our mind, which, by stimulating the same opiate receptors, make us feel happy and satisfied.

Now by stopping them and losing this stimulus, it may happen that, on the contrary, we feel a little sad and nervous.

Many are frightened of these symptoms and not being well informed. They believe that the ketogenic diet is not for them, that they are worse than when they started and abandon everything before going all the way to ketosis.

Running into deficiencies in salts and minerals

A possible lack of minerals can exacerbate the desire for sugars that are accused at the beginning. It is, therefore, necessary to integrate with the right doses of potassium, magnesium, and sodium. Using Himalayan salt, eating salty snacks, using magnesium in the evening could be just as many ways to remedy this mistake.

Consume too much protein

Higher doses of protein help overcome hunger crises, but it is good to go back to consuming the right amount.

To find out how many proteins to consume, just multiply your body weight by 0.8 (if you make a regular physical effort) or 1.2 (if you are a sportsman).

Another common mistake is to consume poor-quality proteins, such as pork and cold cuts.

Insufficient fat consumption

This is another mistake that is easy to run into if we follow the ketogenic diet. We continue to be afraid of consuming fats and not using all-natural sources: coconut oil, ghee, MCT oil, egg yolk, and fatty fish, and butter, avocado. The opposite mistake is to exaggerate with oilseeds: walnuts, almonds, flax seeds, pumpkin seeds. If we neglect to soak in advance with water and lemon, we also absorb the physic acid they contain, a pro substance inflammatory and antinutrient.

Consume bad quality food

It is another of the most common mistakes. We focus on weight loss, but continue to consume frozen, canned, highly processed food and, as mentioned, proteins that are practical and quick to eat but of low quality.

Do not introduce the right amount of fiber

Vegetables should always be fresh, consumed in twice the amount of protein, and always cooked intelligently, never subjected to overcooking or too high temperatures.

In everyday life, if present, however, we often resort to ready-made, frozen, or packaged vegetables.

Also, concerning fruit, we often resort to the very sugary one; we forget that there are many berries with a low glycemic index: berries, mulberries, goji berries, Inca berries, maqui.

Eat raw vegetables

I know this may surprise you, but consuming large quantities of raw vegetables, centrifuged, cold smoothies, over time slow down digestion, cool it, undermine our ability to transform food and absorb nutrients. Over time, this exposes us to inevitable deficiencies: joint pain, teeth, nails and weak hair, anemia, tiredness, abnormal weight loss.

Consume the highest protein load at dinner

This is a mistake that involuntarily, we all commit. The work, the thousand commitments, leads us to stay out all day, to eat a frugal meal for lunch, or even not to consume it at all. Here the dinner turns into the only moment of the day in which we find our family members. We have more time, we are more relaxed, and we finally allow ourselves a real meal complete with vegetables, proteins, sometimes even carbohydrates, and then fruit or dessert to finish.

It escapes us that even the healthiest protein, the freshest or most organic food, weighs down the liver. During the night, this being busy helping digestion, it cannot perform the other precious task: to purify the blood, prepare hormones, energy for the next day.

Not drinking enough

And above all, don't drink hot water. You got it right. Drinking hot water is another story entirely, a massive difference from drinking it even at room temperature. The benefits are many: more excellent digestibility and absorption, deep hydration of cells, brighter skin and hair, retention disappear, cellulite improves, kidneys are strengthened, digestion improves, heartburn subsides.

So, in conclusion, if you avoid these nine mistakes:

- give up before completing ketosis
- incurring deficiencies in salts and minerals
- consuming too much protein
- consume few fats
- consume lousy quality food
- do not introduce the right amount of fiber
- consume raw vegetables
- introduce the highest protein load in the evening
- do not drink incredibly hot water

That is, to allow the body to enter and exit the state of ketosis, to use fats as energy fuel, but also to burn glucose when we have it available.

FOODS TO EAT AND FOODS TO AVOID

How did most people who worked hard to lose a lot of weight end up getting it all back? Worse, why are some extra pounds usually tackled on, so folks end up weighing even more than before they began the whole diet process?

Many people believe they can eat, lose weight, and that's it! If the loss wasn't as significant as initially hoped, then they assume the same thing the medical establishment thinks; it's their (the dieter's) fault. They return to their pre-diet way of eating out of a sense of failure and eventually gain all that weight back plus a few extras!

Before you judge yourself or others harshly, though, there are several factors in this way of thinking. Our minds were trained to identify where we've gone wrong; we can move to a different way of eating and learning about the food we choose to consume.

So, what makes weight loss so difficult for millions? To answer this question, we need to look at the food industry and our dietary habits over the past decades, and how we have been taught to think about weight gain from the medical establishment and our governments. Over this period, there have been some changes that our manager how and what we eat daily that may contain some clues about what causes the obesity epidemic we are currently facing.

We'll continue with one of the biggest mistakes. The one that led to so much pain, feelings of shame, and embarrassment for the masses of people who worked hard to lose weight just to see each of those hard-lost pounds pile up. Sadly, it is a firm belief that the solution for obesity can be summed up in that essential phrase we all know so well; "Eat less–exercise more." Eat less, walk more. The commonly accepted idea is that for you to lose weight, the total calories consumed must be less than the calories burned. Thus, eat less –move more.

We're in the thinking camp that believes calories matter. However, if you're careful about your macronutrients, you'll automatically get the correct calorie count. They also accept that hormones are essential, so when designing recipes and meal plans for our Speed Keto system, they employ a balanced approach to ensuring insulin development is regulated.

When you are adopting a ketogenic diet,

make sure to take care of the following food groups and combinations—they should not be included in your diet if you want to sustain the ketosis condition that you are bringing the body in.

Foods that are high in sugar, such as coffee, agave, tea, sports drinks, and maple syrup, must not be consumed. Sugar-sweetened foods should also be stopped.

Grains, along with grain-based foods, are prohibited. It covers granola, oats, grain, barley, pasta, and corn.

Some fruits will also be avoided due to their high amount of carbohydrates. Apples, oranges, and bananas are often considered at the top of the list when looking at fruit to avoid a ketogenic diet.

Tuber vegetables and food products made from these vegetables on the market are some of the items you can't eat. This would include carrots and yams, French fries, and potato chips packets.

It's also important to consider the oils you're cooking with. We mentioned earlier that you should consider using olive oil, coconut oil, and avocado oil. Specific oil solutions tend to be high in fat, which may help a ketogenic diet, but these are the dangerous kinds of fats that contribute to inflammation and other problems in the body.

While most people think that a ketogenic diet is restrictive, they will have to start eliminating many of the items they use to consume—the plan can still be rendered tasty and healthy. The goal here is to make sure you understand exactly what items you can include in your diet—and then use your cooking skills and imagination to develop ways to turn certain foods into healthy and balanced meals.

With a ketogenic diet, your consumption of carbs is relatively reduced. However, your intake of healthy fats is enhanced.

Types of items that come within the correct ranges to make them ideal for a ketogenic diet will have fish, such as oysters, mussels, octopus, squid, clams, and mussels.

Fish such as mackerel, tuna, and sardines.

Vegetables low in carbs, such as spinach, Brussels Sprouts, kale, cauliflower, and broccoli.

Cheese Poultry, including chicken and turkey.

Meat products, preferably grass-fed

Avocados Eggs, ideally omega-3-rich types,

Greek yogurt (unsweetened plain yogurt), Cottage cheese A variety of seeds, such as sesame seeds, pumpkin seeds, chia seeds, and linseeds.

Nuts, such as peanuts, macadamia nuts, pecan nuts, walnuts, Brazil nuts, cashews, and pistachio nuts.

In addition to these food options, it is also important to note that, when cooking food, the three types of oil that you should use are avocado oil, coconut oil, and olive oil. Both three of these oils are considered to be rich in healthy fats and weak in unhealthy fats, and will not have a significant impact on your daily intake of carbohydrates.

Foods To Enjoy On The Ketogenic Diet

Different food types are listed here. These food ideas advocate for high-fat content while also labeling other foods and essential vitamins for the body to use.

Foods and Animal Products—Focus on grass-fed or pasture-raised fat cuts of meat and wild-caught fish, avoiding farmed pet foods and processed meats as much as possible. And don't forget the liver made meats!

Beef

Hen

Chicken

Eggs

Goat
Lamb
Pig
Rabbit
Turkey
Venison
Shellfish
Chicken
Cat
Cow
Goat
Lamb
Pork
Rabbit
Turkey
Venison
Salmon

Tuna
Halibut
Cod
Gelatin
Chicken fat
Coconut fat
Duck fat
Ghee
Lard
Tallow
MCT oil
Avocado oil
Macadamia oil
Extra virgin olive oil
Coconut butter
Coconut

Instead of root vegetables and other starchy veggies, you need to be vigilant about carbohydrates in the ketogenic diet, so stick to leafy greens and low-glycemic veggies. I've put avocados in this section because some of us may remember it as a vegetable even though it's a fruit.

- **Artichokes**
- **Asparagus**
- **Avocado**
- **Broccoli**
- **Bell peppers**
- **Cauliflower**
- **Cabbage**
- **Celery**
- **Cucumber**
- **Lettuce**
- **Kohlrabi**
- **Radishes**
- **Zucchini**
- **Okra or ladies' fingers**
- **Seaweed**
- **Tomatoes**
- **Spinach**
- **Watercress**

Dairy Products– If you can handle dairy products, you can add full-fat, raw dairy products in your diet and unpasteurized. Keep in mind that some brands contain lots of sugar that could increase the carb content, so look out for nutrition labels and limit the intake of these items. When possible, go for the full-fat varieties as these are less likely to be used to substitute the fat with sugar.

- **Cottage cheese**
- **Mozzarella cheese**
- **Swiss cheese**
- **Sour cream**
- **Full-fat yogurt**
- **Heavy cream**

Herbs and Spices – Herbs and spices are an excellent way to flavor your foods while adding a moderate amount of calories or carbs.

- **Black pepper**
- **Basil**
- **Cinnamon**
- **Cayenne**
- **Cilantro**
- **Chili powder**
- **Cumin**
- **Curry powder**
- **Garam masala**
- **Ginger**
- **Nutmeg**
- **Garlic**
- **Oregano**
- **Onion**
- **Paprika**
- **Parsley**
- **Rosemary**
- **Sea salt**
- **Sage**
- **Thyme**
- **Turmeric**
- **White pepper**

Beverages: On the ketogenic diet, you can avoid all sweetened drinks, but there are certain drinks that you can still have.

- **Almond milk unsweetened**
- **Bone broth**
- **Cashew milk unsweetened**
- **Coconut milk**
- **Club soda**
- **Coffee**
- **Herbal tea**

Mineral water
Seltzer water
Tea

28 DAY MEAL PLAN

	BREAKFAST	LUNCH	SNACK	DINNER	DESSERT
1	Chai Waffles	Shirmp Alfredo with Cauliflower rice	Keto Trail Mix	Beef Shanks Braised in Red Wine sauce	Cream Cheese and Pumpkin cups
2	Cheesy Broccoli Muffins	BLT Salad	Strawberry fat Bombs	Tangy Coconut Cod	Blueberry Crisp
3	Green Veggie Quiche	Fish Taco Bowl	Zucchini balls with capers and bacon	Sticky Pork Ribs	Keto Chocolate Cake
4	Yogurt Waffles	Cheesy Bacon Ranch	Kale Chips	Scallops with Bacon Sauce	Vanilla Flan
5	Onion Cheese Muffins	Stuffed Onions	Cauliflower Poppers	Indian Buttered Chicken	Lemon Mug Cake
6	Spinach-Mushroom Frittata	Thai Chicken Salad Bowl	Sweet Onion Dip with Veggie Sticks	Herbed Grilled Lamb	Coconut Chia Pudding
7	Fluffy Chocolate Pancakes	Shepperd's Pie	Cheesy Zucchini Triangles	Cajun Lobster Tails	Lemon Coconut Balls
8	Goat Cheese Frittata	Thai Peanut Chicken Skewers	Kale Chips	Beef Wellington	Granny Smith Apple Tart
9	Bacon Artichocke Omelet	BBQ Pulled Beef	Keto Trail mix	Chicken Parmigiana	Almond Milk Panna Cotta
10	Cheesy Breakfast Muffin	Greek Tuna Salad	Blueberry fat Bombs	Sesame Pork with Green Beans	Green Tea and Macadamia Brownies
11	Chai Waffles	Cheesy CauliFlower Falafel	Herbed Cheese Chips	Lamb Chops with Tapenade	Lemon Almond Coconut Cake
12	Spinach Mushrooms + Goat Cheese Frittata	Israeli Salmon Salad	Keto Trail mix	Swedish Meatballs	Coconut Chia Pudding
13	Berry Chocolate Breakfast Bowl	Chicken Quesadilla	Kale Chips	Keto Red Curry	Strawberry Mousse
14	Coconut - Granola with Almond Milk	Vegan Sandwich with Tofu and Lettuce slaw	Crispy Parmesan Chips	Shirmp Curry	Chocolate Walnut Cookies
15	Crepes with Lemon-Buttery Syrup	Tangy Coconut Cod	Keto Trail mix	Veggie Greek Moussaka	Mini Blueberry Cheesecake
16	Flaxseed, Maple, Pumpkin Muffin	Creamy Shrimp Salad	Blueberry Fat Bombs	Ground Beef Stroganoff	Almond Shortbread Cookie
17	Apple Pancakes	BeefTaco Salad	Kale Chips	Gouda Cauliflower Casserole	PB & J-Cups
18	Green Shakshuka	Black Bean Veggie Burger	Crispy Parmesan Chips	Fried Shrimp Tails	Chocolate and Strawberry Crepes

19	Spinach Mushroom Frittata	Chicken Potpie	Crispy Parmesan Chips	Sweet and Sour Tempeh	Snickerdoodle Muffins
20	Omelet with Onions and Artichoke	Beef Chili	Tex-Mex Queso Dip with Veggie Sticks	Spinach and Zucchini Lasagna	Cashew and Raspberry Truffles
21	Green Shakshuka	Spicy Shrimp Skewers	Keto Trail mix	Coconut and Lime Steak	Keto Chocolate Cake
22	Goat Cheese Frittata	Tuscan Chicken	Keto Bread	Mexican Casserole with Black Beans	Vanilla Flan
23	Berry Chocolate Breakfast Bowl	Shepherd's Pie	Herbed Cheese Chips	Nut Stuffed Pork Chops	Lemon Mug Cake
24	Cajun Crabmeat Frittata	Cherry Tomato Gratin	Blueberry Fat Bombs	Braised Chicken in Tomato Sauce	Coconut Cheesecake
25	Spinach Mushroom Frittata	Chicken Cauliflower Fried Rice	Crispy Parmesan Chips	Parmesan-Garlic Salmon + Asparagus	Chocolate Pudding
26	Omelet with Onions and Artichoke	Chicken Meatloaf Cups with Pancetta	Keto Trail mix	Pork Chops in Blue Cheese Sauce	Sesame Cookies
27	Yogurt Waffles	Creamy Zoodles	Cold Cuts and Cheese Pinwheels	Turkey Breast with Tomato Olive Salsa	Black Been Brownies
28	Green Veggie> Quiche	Chicken Spinach Salad	Keto Trail mix	Curried Fish with Super Greens	Coconut Chia Pudding

9

SHOPPING LIST

Fruits and Vegetables

Kiwi
Banana
Raspberries
Strawberries
Kohlrabi
Turnip
Habanero pepper
Kale
Cherry tomatoes
Watercress
Bell pepper
Scallion
Fresh cilantro
Chives
Parsley
Broccoli
Strawberries
Blueberries
Mushrooms
Spinach
Celery
Green beans
Onion Kale
Lemon
Pumpkin
Apples
Cauliflower
Lemongrass
Squash
Asparagus
Fresh ginger
Brussel sprouts
Eggplant
Cucumber
Avocado
Lime
Jalapeno
Tomatoes

Herbs and Spices

Sage
White pepper
Bay leaf
Rosemary
Italian seasoning blend
Pepper
Salt
Cinnamon
Ground ginger
Ground cloves
Ground cardamom
Curry powder
Ground cumin
Onion powder
Garlic powder
Dried oregano
Allspice
Mint
Garam masala
Paprika
Turmeric
Thyme
Kosher salt
Ground coriander
Garlic salt
Pink Himalayan salt
Cayenne pepper
Ground nutmeg

Dry Good, Nuts and Grains

Dates
Chia seeds
Poppy seeds
Cranberries
Baking Powder
Almond Flour
Flax Seed Meal
Vanilla whey protein powder
Baking soda
Shredded unsweetened coconut
Sunflower seeds
Pumpkin seeds
Walnuts
Cornstarch
Coconut flour
Xanthan gum
Cocoa powder
Cashew nuts
Flaxseeds
Coconut flakes
Sesame seeds
Pecans
Macadamia
Quinoa
Leeks
Fresh dill
Lettuce
Zucchini
Green chili
Artichoke hearts
Garlic
Spinach
Shallots
Carrots

Condiments and Oil

MCT Oil
Brain octane oil
Balsamic vinegar
Pommery Mustard
White vinegar
Worcestershire sauce
Soy sauce
Sriracha sauce
Olive oil
Apple cider vinegar
Mayonnaise
Dijon mustard
Red wine vinegar
Fish sauce
Soy sauce
Almond oil
Avocado oil
Coconut oil
Hot sauce
Coconut aminos

Dairy, cheese and non-dairy substitutes

Buttermilk
Fontina cheese
Crème fraiche
Swiss cheese
Gouda cheese
Gorgonzola cheese
Blue cheese
Queso fresco
Whipping cream
Almond milk
Greek yogurt
Mozzarella cheese
Parmesan cheese
Swiss cheese
Feta cheese
Soy milk
Coconut milk
Ghee
Butter
Fresh Eggs
Cream Cheese
Heavy Whipping Cream
Shredded Mexican Blend Cheese
Colby jack cheese
Sour cream
Goat Cheese
Feta cheese
Mascarpone cheese
Halloumi cheese
Cheddar cheese

Sweeteners and flavorings

Honey
Truvia
Swerve
Almond extract
Cane sugar
Vanilla extract
Chocolate chips
Xylitol
Brown sugar
Maple syrup
Erythritol
Vanilla extract
Liquid stevia
Chocolate buttons
Monk fruit sweetener

Grocery Items

Tahini
Green tea powder
Gelatin powder
Instant coffee
Horseradish
Shirataki noodles
Chickpeas in can
Red curry paste
Coconut cream
Vegetable broth
Pineapple juice
Sugar-free ketchup
Peanut butter
Kalamata olives
Tomato sauce in can
Ranch seasoning
Taco seasoning
Sun-dried tomatoes
Tomato paste
Crushed tomatoes in can
Coleslaw cabbage mix
Chicken broth
Green olives
Tajin chili lime seasoning
Tuna in can
Pumpkin pie spice
Black olives
Cajun seasoning
Soft/silken tofu
Frozen peas
Dill relish
Dill pickles
Black beans in can
Corn tortillas
Pork rinds
Firm tofu
Liver pate
Beef broth
Sugar-free BBQ sauce
Liquid smoke

Meat and Cold-cuts

Salami
Pepperoncini
Turkey sausage
Skirt steak
Pork butt roast
French-cut lamb chops
Chuck roast
Pork chops
Pork loin roast
Pork ribs
Beef tenderloin steaks
Beef shanks
Lamb
Ground pork
Pancetta
Ground beef
Turkey
Chicken thighs
Turkey ham
Prosciutto
Chicken breast
Bacon

Seafood

Cod fillets
Tilapia fillets
Crabmeat
Smoked salmon
Sea bass fillets
Mahi-mahi fillers
Fresh salmon
Mackerel fillets
Clams or mussels
Halibut fillets
Shrimps
Scallops
Lobster

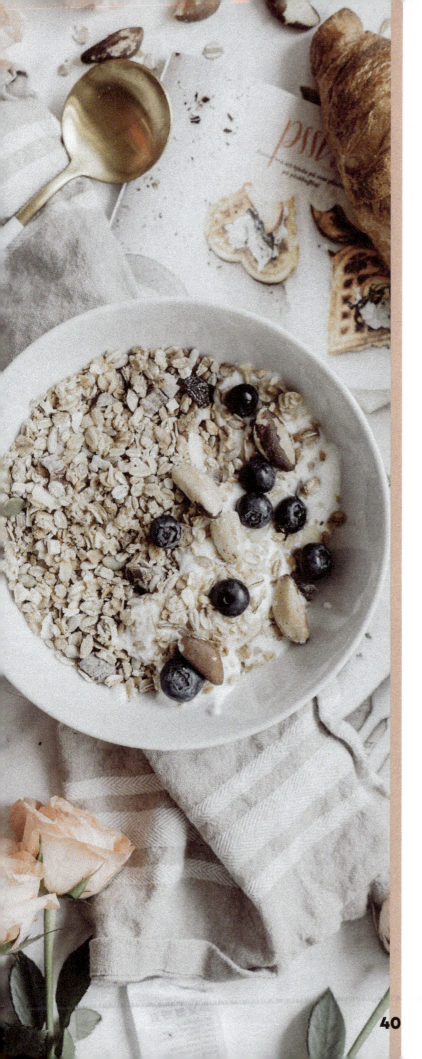

BREAKFAST RECIPES

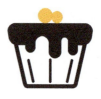

CHEESY BREAKFAST MUFFINS

Prep Time: 15 min   **Cooking Time:** 12 min   **Servings:** 6

Ingredients:

Ingredients:

- 4 tablespoons melted butter
- 3/4 tablespoon baking powder
- 1 cup almond flour
- 2 large eggs, lightly beaten
- 2 ounces cream cheese mixed with 2 tablespoons heavy whipping cream
- A handful of shredded Mexican blend cheese

Directions:

Directions:

1. Preheat the oven to 400°F. Grease 6 muffin tin cups with melted butter and set aside.
2. Combine the baking powder and almond flour in a bowl. Stir well and set aside.
3. Stir together four tablespoons melted butter, eggs, shredded cheese, and cream cheese in a separate bowl.
4. The egg and the dry mixture must be combined using a hand mixer to beat until it is creamy and well blended.
5. The mixture must be scooped into the greased muffin cups evenly.

Nutrition:
Calories: 214kcal   **Fat:** 15.6   **Fiber:** 3.1g   **Carbohydrates:** 5.1g   **Protein:** 9.5 g

YOGURT WAFFLES

Prep Time: 15 min   **Cooking time:** 25 min   **Servings:** 5

Ingredients:

- 1/2 cup golden flax seeds meal
- 1/2 cup plus 3 tablespoons almond flour
- 1-1 1/2 tablespoons granulated Erythritol
- 1 tablespoon unsweetened vanilla whey protein powder
- 1/4 teaspoon baking soda
- 1/2 teaspoon organic baking powder
- 1/4 teaspoon xanthan gum
- Salt, as required
- 1 large organic egg, white and yolk separated
- 1 organic whole egg
- 2 tablespoons unsweetened almond milk
- 1 1/2 tablespoons unsalted butter
- 3 ounces plain Greek yogurt

Directions:

1. Preheat the waffle iron and then grease it.
2. In a large bowl, add the flour, Erythritol, protein powder, baking soda, baking powder, xanthan gum, salt, and mix until well combined.
3. In another bowl or container, put in the egg white and beat until stiff peaks form.
4. In a third bowl, add two egg yolks, whole egg, almond milk, butter, yogurt, and beat until well combined.
5. Place egg mixture into the bowl of the flour mixture and mix until well combined.
6. Gently, fold in the beaten egg whites.
7. Place 1/4 cup of the mixture into preheated waffle iron and cook for about 4–5 minutes or until golden brown.
8. Repeat with the remaining mixture.
9. Serve warm.

Nutrition:
Calories: 265kcal   **Fat:** 11.5   **Fiber:** 9.5g   **Carbohydrates:** 5.2g   **Protein:** 7.5 g

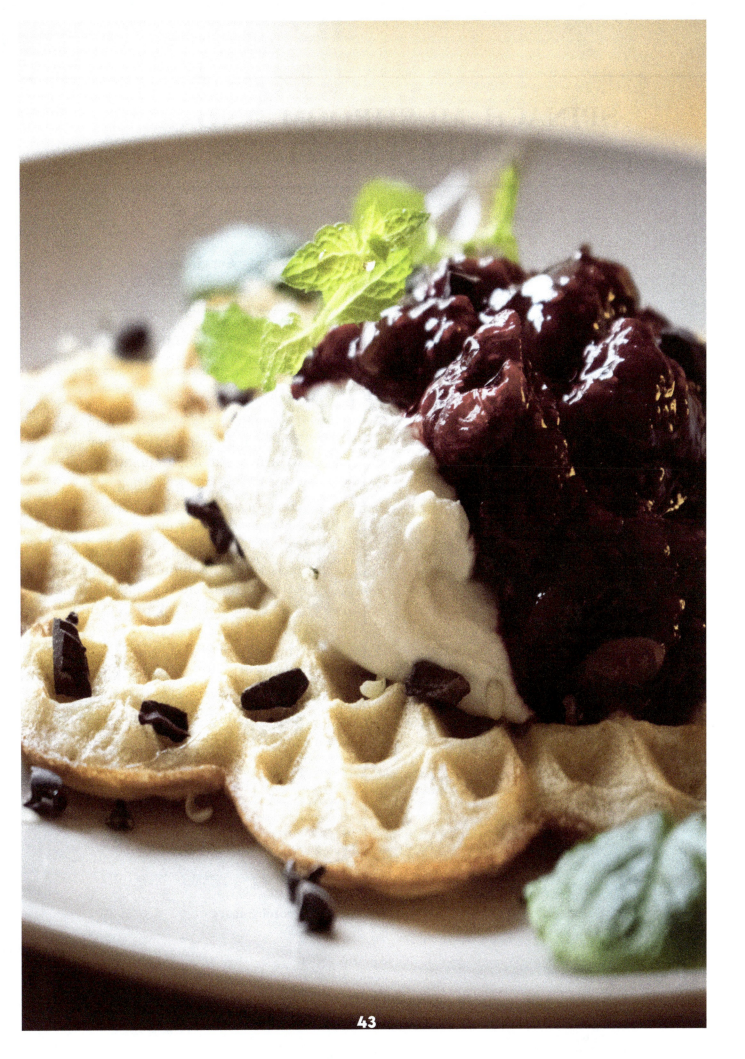

SPINACH, MUSHROOM, AND GOAT CHEESE FRITTATA

Prep Time: 15 min   **Cooking time:** 20 min   **Servings:** 5

Ingredients:

- 2 tablespoons olive oil
- 1 cup fresh mushrooms, sliced
- 6 bacon slices, cooked and chopped
- 1 cup spinach, shredded
- 10 large eggs, beaten
- 1/2 cup goat cheese, crumbled
- Pepper and salt

Directions:

1. Preheat the oven to 350°F.
2. Heat oil and add the mushrooms and fry for 3 minutes until they start to brown, stirring frequently.
3. Fold in the bacon and spinach and cook for about 1 to 2 minutes, or until the spinach is wilted.
4. Slowly pour in the beaten eggs and cook for 3 to 4 minutes. Making use of a spatula, lift the edges for allowing uncooked egg to flow underneath.
5. Top with the goat cheese, then sprinkle the salt and pepper to season.
6. Bake in the preheated oven for about 15 minutes until lightly golden brown around the edges.

Nutrition:
Calories: 265kcal   **Fat:** 11.6   **Fiber:** 8.6g   **Carbohydrates:** 5.1g   **Protein:** 12.9 g

CHEESY BROCCOLI MUFFINS

Prep Time: 15 min   **Cooking time:** 20 min   **Servings:** 6

Ingredients:

- 2 tablespoons unsalted butter
- 6 large organic eggs
- 1/2 cup heavy whipping cream
- 1/2 cup Parmesan cheese, grated
- Salt and ground black pepper, as required
- 1 1/4 cups broccoli, chopped
- 2 tablespoons fresh parsley, chopped
- 1/2 cup Swiss cheese, grated

Directions:

1. Grease a 12-cup muffin tin.
2. In a bowl or container, put in the cream, eggs, Parmesan cheese, salt, and black pepper, and beat until well combined.
3. Divide the broccoli and parsley in the bottom of each prepared muffin cup evenly.
4. Top with the egg mixture, followed by the Swiss cheese.
5. Let the muffins bake for about 20 minutes, rotating the pan once halfway through.
6. Carefully, invert the muffins onto a serving platter and serve warm.

Nutrition:
Calories: 241kcal   Fat: 11.5   Fiber: 8.5g   Carbohydrates: 4.1g   Protein: 11.1 g

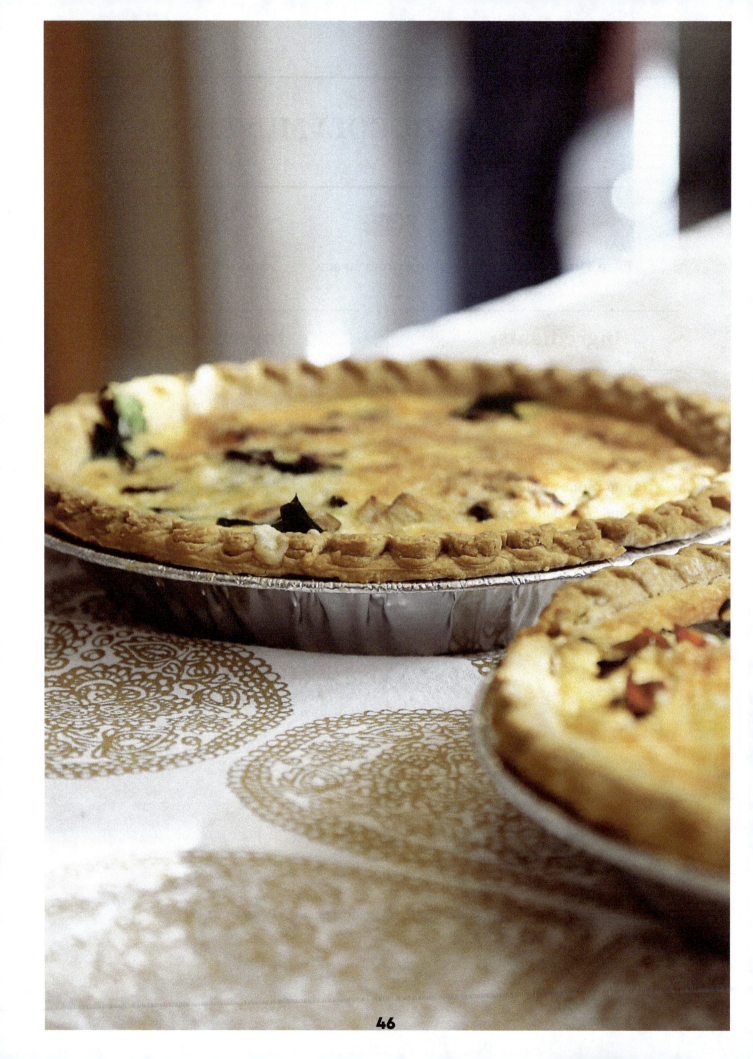

GREEN VEGETABLE QUICHE

Prep Time: 20 min   **Cooking time:** 20 min   **Servings:** 4

Ingredients:

- 6 organic eggs
- 1/2 cup unsweetened almond milk
- Salt and ground black pepper, as required
- 2 cups fresh baby spinach, chopped
- 1/2 cup green bell pepper, seeded and chopped
- 1 scallion, chopped
- 1/4 cup fresh cilantro, chopped
- 1 tablespoon fresh chives, minced
- 3 tablespoons mozzarella cheese, grated

Directions:

1. Preheat your oven to 400°F.
2. Lightly grease a pie dish.
3. In a bowl, add eggs, almond milk, salt, and black pepper, and beat until well combined. Set aside.
4. In another bowl, add the vegetables and herbs and mix well.
5. At the bottom of the prepared pie dish, place the veggie mixture evenly and top with the egg mixture.
6. Let the quiche bake for about 20 minutes.
7. Remove the pie dish from the oven and immediately sprinkle with the Parmesan cheese.
8. Set aside for about 5 minutes before slicing.
9. Cut into desired sized wedges and serve warm.

Nutrition:
Calories: 298kcal   **Fat:** 10.4   **Fiber:** 5.9g   **Carbohydrates:** 4.1g   **Protein:** 7.9 g

BERRY CHOCOLATE BREAKFAST

Prep Time: 10 min   **Cooking time:** 0 min   **Servings:** 2

Ingredients:

- 1/2 cup strawberries, fresh or frozen
- 1/2 cup blueberries, fresh or frozen
- 1 cup unsweetened almond milk
- Sugar-free maple syrup to taste
- 2 tbsp. unsweetened cocoa powder
- 1 tbsp. cashew nuts for topping

Directions:

1. The berries must be divided into four bowls, pour on the almond milk.
2. Drizzle with the maple syrup and sprinkle the cocoa powder on top, a tablespoon per bowl.
3. Top with the cashew nuts and enjoy immediately.

Nutrition:
Calories: 287kcal   Fat: 5.9   Fiber: 11.4g   Carbohydrates: 3.1g   Protein: 4.2 g

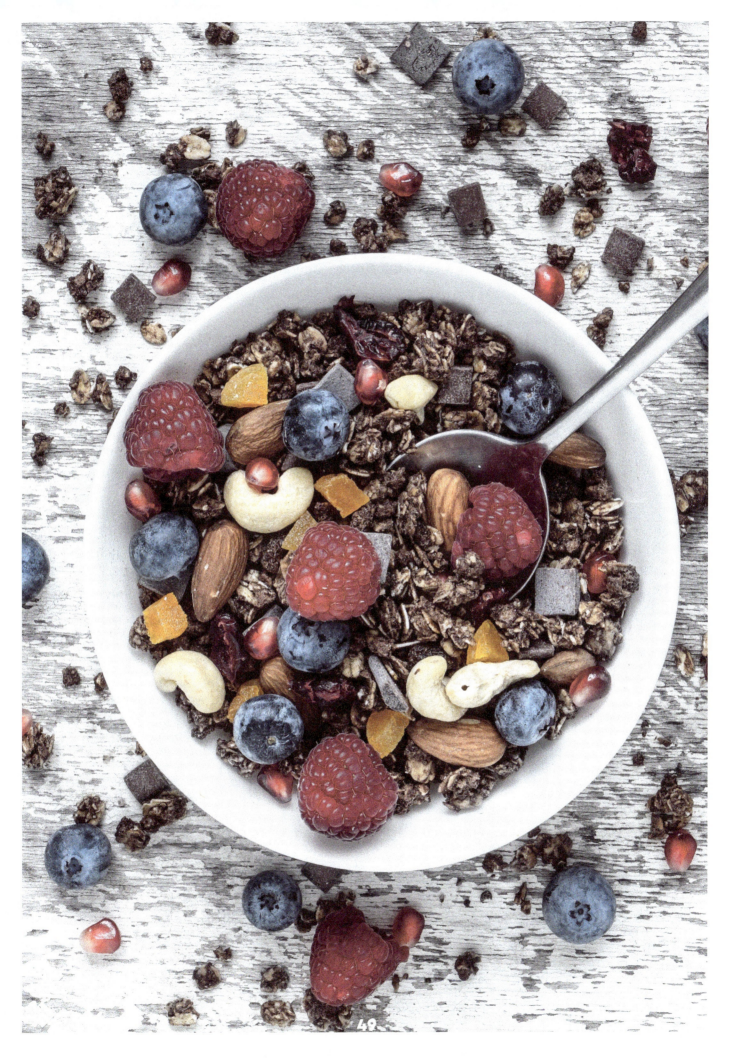

GOAT CHEESE FRITTATA

Prep Time: 15 min   **Cooking time:** 15 min   **Servings:** 4

Ingredients:

- 1 tbsp. avocado oil for frying
- 2 oz. (56 g) bacon slices, chopped
- 1 red bell pepper
- 1 small yellow onion, chopped
- 2 scallions, chopped
- 1 tbsp. chopped fresh chives
- Salt and black pepper to taste
- 8 eggs, beaten
- 1 tbsp. unsweetened almond milk
- 1 tbsp. chopped fresh parsley
- 3 1/2 oz. (100 g) goat cheese, divided
- 3/4 oz. (20 g) grated Parmesan cheese

Directions:

1. Let the oven preheat to 350°F/175°C.
2. Heat the avocado oil in a medium cast-iron pan and cook the bacon for 5 minutes or golden brown. Stir in the bell pepper, onion, scallions, and chives.
3. Cook for 3 to 4 minutes or until the vegetables soften. Season with salt and black pepper.
4. In a bowl or container, the eggs must be beaten with the almond milk and parsley.
5. Pour the mixture over the vegetables, stirring to spread out nicely. Share half of the goat cheese on top.
6. Once the eggs start to set, divide the remaining goat cheese on top, season with salt, black pepper, and place the pan in the oven—Bake for 5 to 6 minutes or until the eggs set all around.
7. Take out the pan, scatter the Parmesan cheese on top, slice, and serve warm.

Nutrition:
Calories: 412kcal   **Fat:** 15.4   **Fiber:** 11.2g   **Carbohydrates:** 4.9g   **Protein:** 10.5 g

GREEN SHAKSHUKA

Prep Time: 15 min   **Cooking time:** 10 min   **Servings:** 4

Ingredients:

- 1 tbsp. olive oil
- 2 tbsp. almond oil
- 1/2 medium green bell pepper, deseeded and chopped
- 1 celery stalk, chopped
- 1/4 cup (57 g) green beans, chopped
- 1 garlic clove, minced
- 2 tbsp. fresh mint leaves
- 3 tbsp. fresh parsley leaves
- 1/2 cup (113 g) baby kale
- 1/4 tsp. plain vinegar
- Salt and black pepper to taste
- 1/4 tsp. nutmeg powder
- 7 oz. (200 g) feta cheese, divided
- 4 eggs

Directions:

1. Heat the olive oil and almond oil in a medium frying pan over medium heat.
2. Add the bell pepper, celery, green beans, and sauté for 5 minutes or until the vegetables soften.
3. Stir in the garlic, mint leaves, two tablespoons of parsley, and cook until fragrant, 1 minute.
4. Add the kale, vinegar, and mix. Once the kale starts wilting, season with salt, black pepper, nutmeg powder, and stir in half of the feta cheese—Cook for 1 to 2 minutes.
5. After, use the spatula to create four holes in the food and crack an egg into each hole. Cook until the egg whites set still running.
6. Season the eggs with salt and black pepper.
7. Turn the heat off and scatter the remaining feta cheese on top.
8. Garnish with the remaining parsley and serve the shakshuka immediately.

Nutrition:
Calories: 322kcal   **Fat:** 14.1   **Fiber:** 10.3g   **Carbohydrates:** 9.4g   **Protein:** 13.1 g

FLUFFY CHOCOLATE PANCAKES

Prep Time: 15 min   **Cooking time:** 12 min   **Servings:** 4

Ingredients:

- 2 cups (250 g) almond flour
- 2 tsp. baking powder
- 2 tbsp... Erythritol
- 3/4 tsp. salt
- 2 eggs
- 1 1/3 cups (320 ml) almond milk
- 2 tbsp. butter + more for frying
- Topping:
- 2 tbsp. unsweetened chocolate buttons
- Sugar-free maple syrup
- 4 tbsp. semi-salted butter

Directions:

1. In a bowl or container, mix the almond flour, baking powder, Erythritol, and salt.
2. Whisk the eggs, almond milk, and butter in another bowl.
3. Combine in the dry ingredients and mix well.
4. Melt about 1 1/2 tablespoon of butter in a non-stick skillet, pour in portions of the batter to make small circles, about two pieces per batch (approximately 1/4 cup of batter each).
5. Sprinkle some chocolate buttons on top and cook for 1 to 2 minutes or until set beneath.
6. Turn the pancakes and cook for one more minute or until set.
7. Remove the pancakes onto a plate and make more with the remaining ingredients.
8. Work with more butter and reduce the heat as needed to prevent sticking and burning.
9. Drizzle the pancakes with some maple syrup, top with more butter (as desired), and enjoy!

Nutrition:
Calories: 384kcal   **Fat:** 12.9   **Fiber:** 5.4g   **Carbohydrates:** 7.5g   **Protein:** 11.9 g

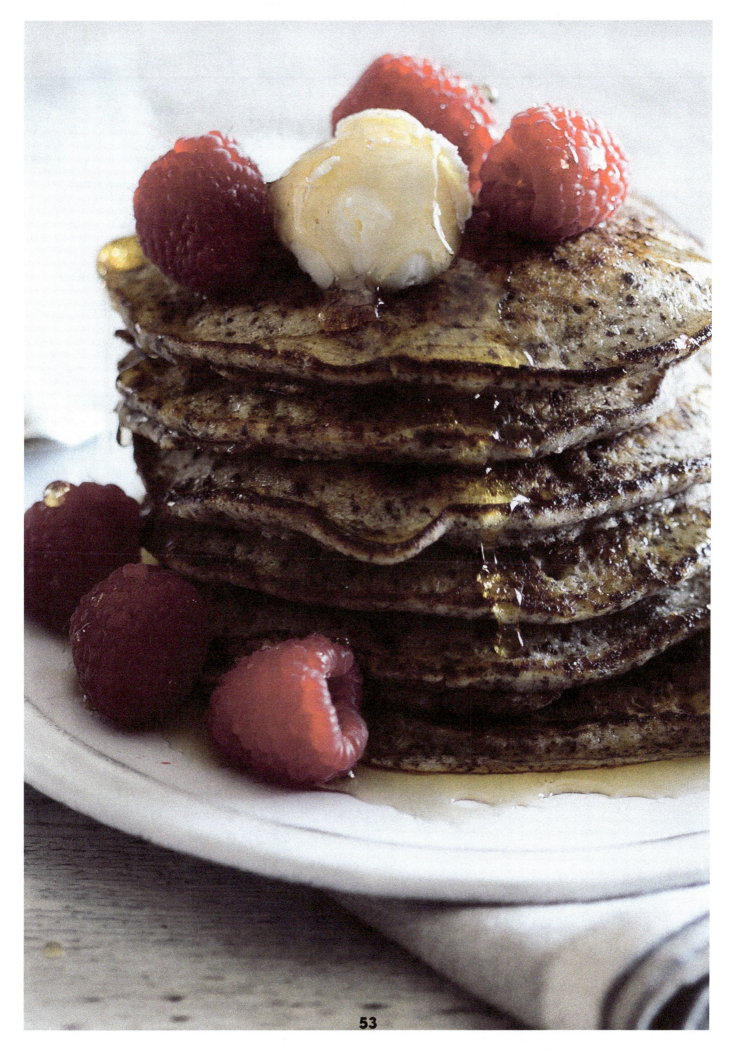

CHAI WAFFLES

Prep Time: 15 min **Cooking time:** 20 min **Servings:** 4

Ingredients:

- 4 eggs, separated
- 3 tablespoons coconut flour
- 3 tablespoons powdered Erythritol
- 1 1/4 teaspoon baking powder
- 1 teaspoon vanilla extract
- 1/2 teaspoon ground cinnamon
- 1/4 teaspoon ground ginger
- Pinch ground cloves
- Pinch ground cardamom
- 3 tablespoons coconut oil, melted
- 3 tablespoons unsweetened almond milk

Directions:

1. Divide the eggs into two separate mixing bowls.
2. Whip the whites until stiff peaks develop and then set aside.
3. Whisk the egg yolks into the other bowl with the coconut flour, Erythritol, baking powder, cocoa, cinnamon, cardamom, and cloves.
4. Pour the melted coconut oil and the almond milk into the second bowl and whisk.
5. Fold softly in the whites of the egg until you have just combined.
6. Preheat waffle iron with cooking spray and grease.
7. Spoon into the iron for about 1/2 cup of batter.
8. Cook the waffle according to directions from the maker.
9. Move the waffle to a plate and repeat with the batter leftover.

Nutrition:
Calories: 286kcal **Fat:** 13.9 **Fiber:** 8.5g **Carbohydrates:** 4.8g **Protein:** 12.8 g

"COCO-NUT" GRANOLA

Prep Time: 10 min   **Cooking time:** 60 min   **Servings:** 8

Ingredients:

- 2 cups shredded unsweetened coconut
- 1 cup sliced almonds
- 1 cup raw sunflower seeds
- 1/2 cup raw pumpkin seeds
- 1/2 cup walnuts
- 1/2 cup melted coconut oil
- 10 drops liquid stevia
- 1 teaspoon ground cinnamon
- 1/2 teaspoon ground nutmeg

Directions:

1. Preheat the oven to 250°F. Line 2 baking sheets with parchment paper. Set aside.
2. Toss all the ingredients together.
3. The granola will then put into baking sheets and spread it out evenly.
4. Bake the granola for about 1 hr.

Nutrition:
Calories: 131kcal   **Fat:** 4.1   **Fiber:** 5.8g   **Carbohydrates:** 2.8g   **Protein:** 5.6 g

BACON ARTICHOKE OMELET

Prep Time: 10 min   **Cooking time:** 10 min   **Servings:** 4

Ingredients:

- 6 eggs, beaten
- 2 tablespoons heavy (whipping) cream
- 8 bacon slices, cooked and chopped
- 1 tablespoon olive oil
- 1/4 cup chopped onion
- 1/2 cup chopped artichoke hearts (canned, packed in water)
- Sea salt
- Freshly ground black pepper

Directions:

1. In a bowl or container, the eggs, heavy cream, and bacon must be mixed.
2. Heat olive oil then sauté the onion until tender, about 3 minutes.
3. Pour the egg mixture into the skillet for 1 minute.
4. Cook the omelet, lifting the edges with a spatula to let the uncooked egg flow underneath, for 2 minutes.
5. Sprinkle the artichoke hearts on top and flip the omelet.
6. Cook for 4 minutes more until the egg is firm.
7. Flip the omelet over again, so the artichoke hearts are on top.
8. Remove from the heat, cut the omelet into quarters, and season with salt and black pepper.
9. Transfer the omelet to plates and serve.

Nutrition:
Calories: 314kcal   **Fat:** 7.1   **Fiber:** 5.4g   **Carbohydrates:** 3.1g   **Protein:** 8.5 g

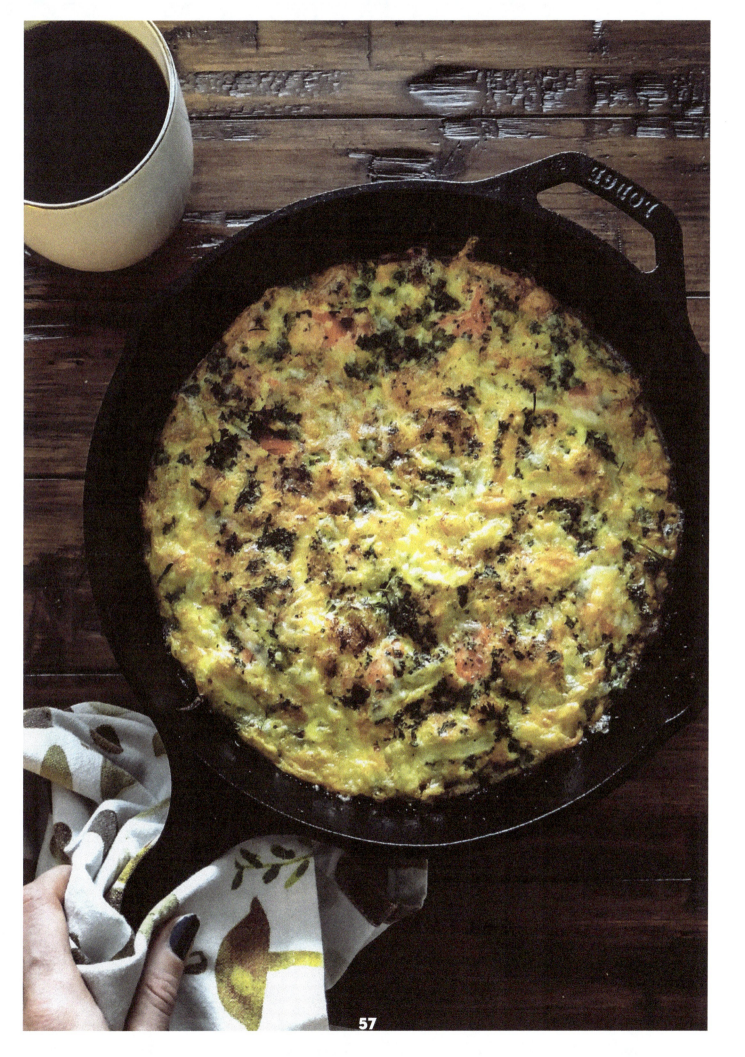

SPINACH-MUSHROOM FRITTATA

Prep Time: 10 min **Cooking time:** 15 min **Servings:** 6

Ingredients:

- 2 tablespoons olive oil
- 1 cup sliced fresh mushrooms
- 1 cup shredded spinach
- 6 bacon slices, cooked and chopped
- 10 large eggs, beaten
- 1/2 cup crumbled goat cheese
- Sea salt
- Freshly ground black pepper

Directions:

1. Preheat the oven to 350°F.
2. Heat olive oil and sauté the mushrooms until lightly browned about 3 minutes.
3. Add the spinach and bacon and sauté until the greens are wilted about 1 minute.
4. Add the eggs and cook, lifting the edges of the frittata with a spatula so uncooked egg flow underneath, for 3 to 4 minutes.
5. Sprinkle with crumbled goat cheese and season lightly with salt and pepper.
6. Bake until set and lightly browned, about 15 minutes.
7. Remove the frittata from the oven, and let it stand for 5 minutes.
8. Cut into six wedges and serve immediately.

Nutrition:
Calories: 312kcal **Fat:** 6.8 **Fiber:** 5.1g **Carbohydrates:** 3.1g **Protein:** 10.5 g

CRÊPES WITH LEMON-BUTTERY

Prep Time: 15 min   **Cooking time:** 20 min   **Servings:** 6

Ingredients:

- 6 ounces mascarpone cheese, softened
- 6 eggs
- 1 1/2 tbsp. granulated swerve
- 1/4 cup almond flour
- 1 tsp. baking soda
- 1 tsp. baking powder
- For the Syrup
- 3/4 cup of water
- 2 tbsp. lemon juice
- 1 tbsp. butter
- 3/4 cup swerve, powdered
- 1 tbsp. vanilla extract
- 1/2 tsp. xanthan gum

Directions:

1. With the use of an electric mixer, mix all crepes ingredients until well incorporated.
2. Use melted butter to grease a frying pan and set over medium heat; cook the crepes.
3. Flip over and cook the other side for a further 2 minutes; repeat the remaining batter.
4. Put the crepes on a plate.
5. In the same pan, mix swerve, butter and water; simmer for 6 minutes as you stir.
6. Transfer the mixture to a blender and a 1/4 teaspoon of xanthan gum and vanilla extract and mix well.
7. Place in the remaining 1/4 teaspoon of xanthan gum and allow to sit until the syrup is thick.

Nutrition:
Calories: 312kcal   **Fat:** 11.5   **Fiber:** 3.8g   **Carbohydrates:** 2.4g   **Protein:** 5.1 g

FLAXSEED, MAPLE & PUMPKIN

Prep Time: 10 min   **Cooking time:** 30 min   **Servings:** 6

Ingredients:

- 1 tbsp. cinnamon
- 1 cup pure pumpkin puree
- 1 tbsp. pumpkin pie spice
- 2 tbsp. coconut oil
- 1 egg
- 1/2 tbsp. baking powder
- 1/2 tsp. salt
- 1/2 tsp. apple cider vinegar
- 1/2 tsp. vanilla extract
- 1/3 cup erythritol
- 1 1/4 cup flaxseeds (ground)
- 1/4 cup Maple Syrup

Directions:

1. Line ten muffin tins with ten muffin liners and preheat oven to 350oF.
2. All the ingredients must be blended until smooth and creamy, around 5 minutes.
3. Evenly divide batter into prepared muffin tins.
4. Pop in the oven and let it bake for 20 minutes or until tops are lightly browned.
5. Let it cool. Evenly divide into suggested servings and place in meal prep containers.

Nutrition:
Calories: 241kcal   **Fat:** 11.3   **Fiber:** 15.9g   **Carbohydrates:** 3.1g   **Protein:** 8.9g

ONION CHEESE MUFFINS

Prep Time: 15 min **Cooking time:** 20 min **Servings:** 6

Ingredients:

- 1/4 cup Colby jack cheese, shredded
- 1/4 cup shallots, minced
- 1/2 tsp. salt
- 1 cup almond flour
- 1 egg
- 3 tbsp. melted butter
- 3 tbsp. sour cream

Directions:

1. Line 6 muffin tins with six muffin liners. Set aside and preheat oven to 350°F.
2. In a bowl, stir the dry and wet ingredients alternately. Mix well.
3. Scoop a spoonful of the batter to the prepared muffin tins.
4. Bake for 20 minutes in the oven until golden brown.

Nutrition:
Calories: 241kcal **Fat:** 5.1 **Fiber:** 2.6g **Carbohydrates:** 3.1g **Protein:** 4.2 g

CAJUN CRABMEAT FRITTATA

Prep Time: 15 min   **Cooking time:** 20 min   **Servings:** 4

Ingredients:

- 1 tbsp. olive oil
- 1 onion, chopped
- 4 ounces crabmeat, chopped
- 1 tsp. Cajun seasoning
- 6 large eggs, slightly beaten
- 1/2 cup Greek yogurt

Directions:

1. Let the oven preheat to 350°F/175°C, then set a large skillet over medium heat and warm the oil.
2. Add in onion and sauté until soft; place in crabmeat and cook for two more minutes.
3. Season with Cajun seasoning.
4. Evenly distribute the ingredients at the bottom of the skillet.
5. Whisk the eggs with yogurt.
6. Transfer to the skillet.
7. Put it in the oven and let the frittata bake for about 18 minutes or until eggs are cooked.
8. Slice into wedges and serve warm.

Nutrition:
Calories: 256kcal   **Fat:** 4.9   **Fiber:** 2.9g   **Carbohydrates:** 3.1g   **Protein:** 8.9g

OMELET WITH ONIONS AND ARTICHOKE

Prep Time: 15 min   **Cooking time:** 20 min   **Servings:** 4

Ingredients:

- 6 eggs, beaten until frothy
- 2 tbsp. whipped cream
- 8 slices of bacon, cooked and chopped
- 1 tbsp. olive oil
- 1/4 cup chopped onions
- 1/2 cup chopped artichoke hearts (canned)
- sea-salt
- Freshly ground black pepper

Directions:

1. Mix the eggs, whipped cream, and bacon in a small bowl and set aside.
2. Heat olive oil then steam the onions gently (approx. 3 minutes).
3. The mixture must be poured into the pan and stir for 1 minute.
4. Cook the omelet and lift the edges with a spatula so that the uncooked egg can flow under the omelet (approx. 2 minutes).
5. Scatter the artichoke hearts on top and turn the omelet. Cook for another 4 minutes until the egg is firm.
6. Turn the omelet again so that the artichoke hearts are on top.
7. Remove from heat, quarter the omelet, and season with salt and black pepper.
8. Serve hot.

Nutrition:
Calories: 312kcal   **Fat:** 14   **Fiber:** 11g   **Carbohydrates:** 3.1g   **Protein:** 9.5g

APPLE PANCAKES

Prep Time: 15 min   **Cooking time:** 25 min   **Servings:** 4

Ingredients:

- 2 chopped apples
- 1/2 cup of soft/silken Tofu
- 1/3 cup of vegetable shortening
- 1 1/2 cups of soy milk
- 2 1/2 teaspoons of baking powder
- 1 1/2 cups of almond flour
- 1/2 teaspoon of cinnamon
- 1/2 teaspoon of nutmeg
- 1/3 cup of chopped pecans
- 2 tablespoons of olive oil

Directions:

1. Get a blender or food processor. Put the chopped apples, soft tofu, vegetable, flour, baking powder, and soy milk.
2. Blend everything until it's well blended. Add the nutmeg, cinnamon to the mixture.
3. Blend again until the apples are well minced, and all the ingredients are incorporated and blended.
4. Pick the pecans and gently fold the blended ingredients in the pecans.
5. Prepare a large skillet by oiling it.
6. Use a large spoon; take a spoonful of the pecans and drop in the skillet.
7. Cook the pecans until bubbles appear; this usually takes a few minutes.
8. Flip the pecan to the other side and cook until both sides are lightly golden brown.
9. Serve and enjoy!

Nutrition:
Calories: 298kcal   **Fat:** 11.4   **Fiber:** 3.1g   **Carbohydrates:** 5.2g   **Protein:** 12.9 g

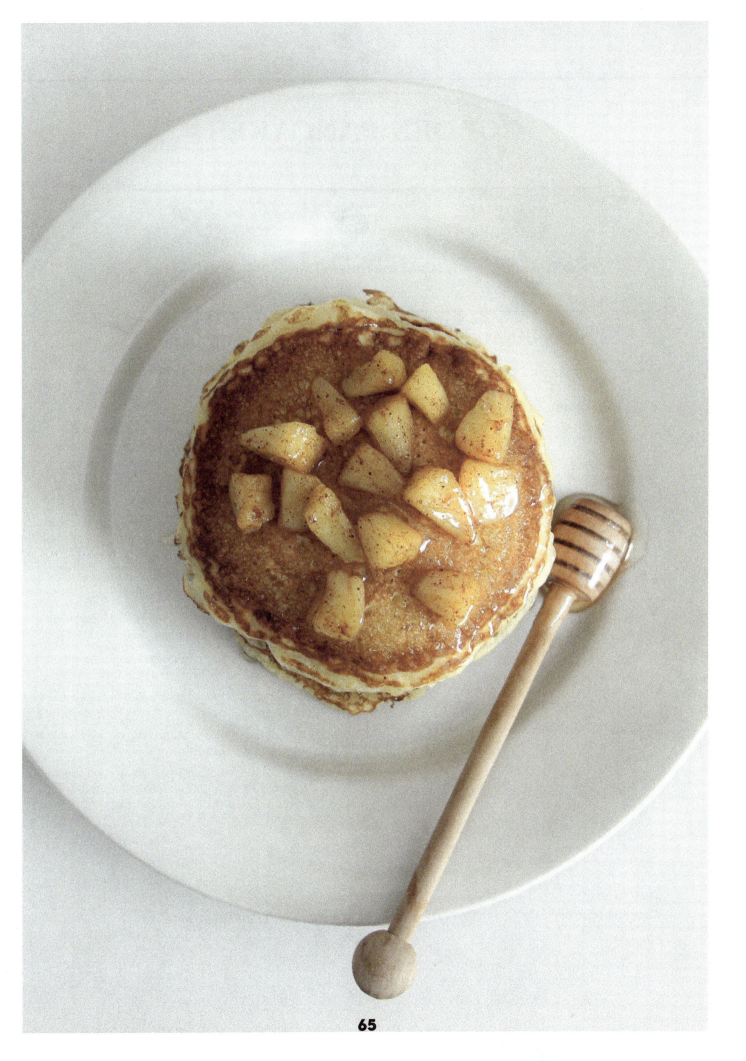

GOLDEN PANCAKES

Prep Time: 5 min   **Cooking time:** 15 min   **Servings:** 4

Ingredients:

- 2/3 cup almond flour
- 1/3 cup coconut flour
- 1 tablespoon monk fruit sweetener, powder form (optional)
- 1 teaspoon baking powder
- 1/4 teaspoon ground nutmeg
- 3 eggs
- 1/4 to 1/2 cup of coconut milk
- 3 tablespoons coconut oil
- 1 teaspoon pure vanilla extract
- Grass-fed butter, for cooking the pancakes
- 1/2 cup sugar-free syrup (optional)

Directions:

1. Mix the dry ingredients.
2. In a large bowl, stir together the almond flour, coconut flour, monk fruit sweetener (if using), baking powder, and nutmeg until everything is well blended.
3. Add the wet ingredients.
4. In a container or bowl, whisk together the eggs, 1/4 cup of the coconut milk, and the coconut oil and vanilla.
5. Add the wet ingredients to the dry ingredients and whisk until the batter is smooth.
6. If the batter is too thick, add more coconut milk.
7. Cook the pancakes. In a pan, melt the butter.
8. Drop the pancake batter by tablespoons, about 3 per pancake, and spread it out to form circles.
9. You should be able to cook about four pancakes per batch.
10. Cook until bubbles form on the pancakes and burst, about 2 minutes.
11. Transfer the pancakes to a plate and set it aside. Repeat with the remaining batter until it's all used up.
12. Serve.

Nutrition:
Calories: 298kcal   **Fat:** 5.1   **Fiber:** 11g   **Carbohydrates:** 1.2g   **Protein:** 1.4 g

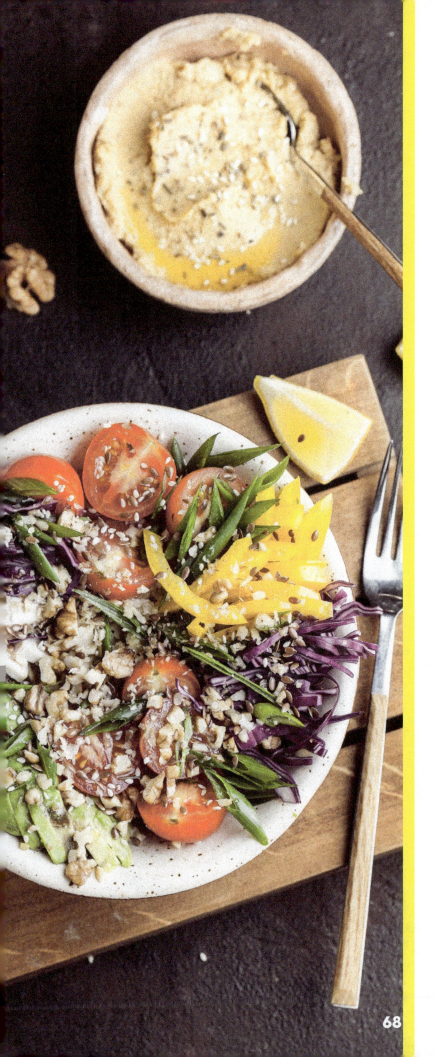

11

APPETIZERS
AND
SIDES

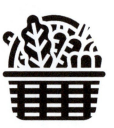

SPICED JALAPENO BITES WITH TOMATO

Prep Time: 10 min   **Cooking time:** 0 min   **Servings:** 4

Ingredients:

- 1 cup turkey ham, chopped
- 1/4 jalapeño pepper, minced
- 1/4 cup mayonnaise
- 1/3 tablespoon Dijon mustard
- 4 tomatoes, sliced
- Salt and black pepper, to taste
- 1 tablespoon parsley, chopped

Directions:

1. In a bowl, mix the turkey ham, jalapeño pepper, mayo, mustard, salt, and pepper.
2. Spread out the tomato slices on four serving plates, then top each plate with a spoonful turkey ham mixture.
3. Serve garnished with chopped parsley.

Nutrition:
Calories: 250kcal   **Fat:** 14.1   **Fiber:** 3.7 g   **Carbohydrates:** 4.2g   **Protein:** 18.9 g

COCONUT CRAB CAKES

Prep Time: 20 min   **Cooking time:** 25 min   **Servings:** 4

Ingredients:

- 1 tablespoon of minced garlic
- 2 pasteurized eggs
- 2 teaspoons of coconut oil
- 3/4 cup of coconut flakes
- 3/4 cup chopped of spinach
- 1/4 pound crabmeat
- 1/4 cup of chopped leek
- 1/2 cup extra virgin olive oil
- 1/2 teaspoon of pepper
- 1/4 onion diced
- Salt

Directions:

1. Pour the crabmeat in a bowl, then add in the coconut flakes and mix well.
2. Whisk eggs in a bowl, then mix in leek and spinach.
3. Season the egg mixture with pepper, two pinches of salt, and garlic.
4. Then, pour the eggs into the crab and stir well.
5. Preheat a pan, heat extra virgin olive, and fry the crab evenly from each side until golden brown. Remove from pan and serve hot.

Nutrition:
Calories: 254kcal   **Fat:** 9.5   **Fiber:** 5.4g   **Carbohydrates:** 4.1g   **Protein:** 8.9 g

TUNA CAKES

Prep Time: 15 min   **Cooking time:** 10 min   **Servings:** 2

Ingredients:

- 1 (15-ounce) can water-packed tuna, drained
- 1/2 celery stalk, chopped
- 2 tablespoon fresh parsley, chopped
- 1 teaspoon fresh dill, chopped
- 2 tablespoons walnuts, chopped
- 2 tablespoons mayonnaise
- 1 organic egg, beaten
- 1 tablespoon butter
- 3 cups lettuce

Directions:

1. For burgers: Add all ingredients (except the butter and lettuce) in a bowl and mix until well combined.
2. Make two equal-sized patties from the mixture.
3. Melt some butter and cook the patties for about 2–3 minutes.
4. Carefully flip the side and cook for about 2–3 minutes.
5. Divide the lettuce onto serving plates.
6. Top each plate with one burger and serve.

Nutrition:
Calories: 267kcal   **Fat:** 12.5   **Fiber:** 9.4g   **Carbohydrates:** 3.8g   **Protein:** 11.5 g

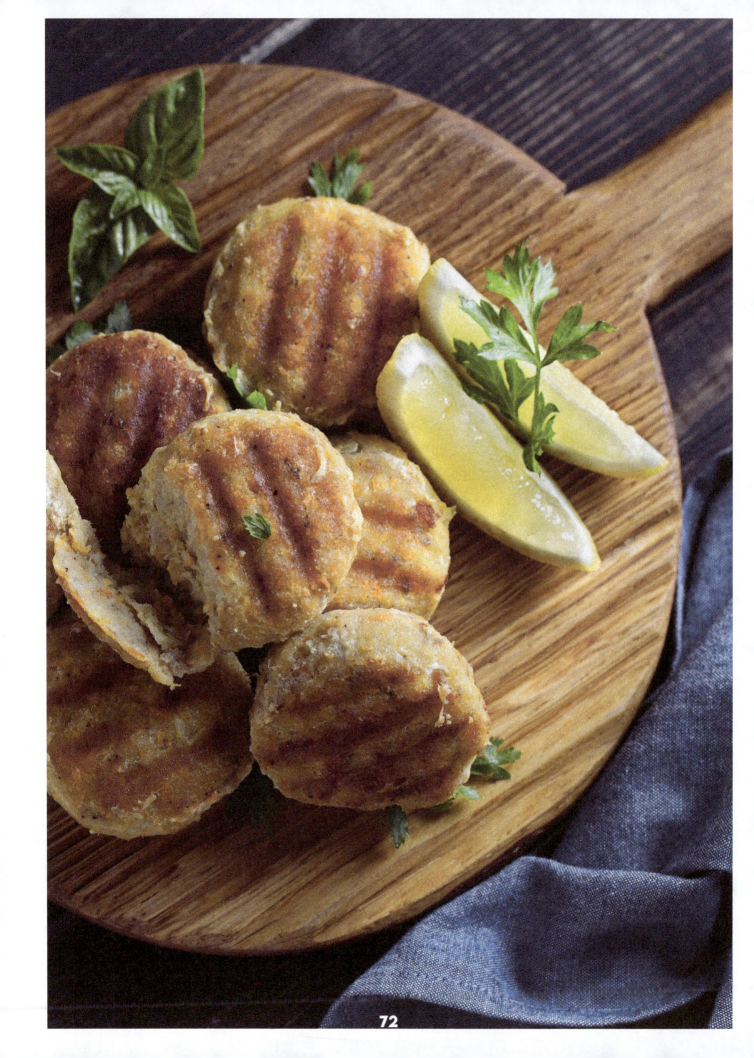

CREAMED SPINACH

Prep Time: 10 min   **Cooking time:** 15 min   **Servings:** 4

Ingredients:

- 2 tablespoons unsalted butter
- 1 small yellow onion, chopped
- 1 cup cream cheese, softened
- 2 (10-ounce) packages frozen spinach, thawed and squeezed dry
- 2–3 tablespoons water
- Salt and ground black pepper, as required
- 1 teaspoon fresh lemon juice

Directions:

1. Melt some butter and sauté the onion for about 6–8 minutes.
2. Add the cream cheese and cook for about 2 minutes or until melted completely.
3. Stir in the water and spinach and cook for about 4–5 minutes.
4. Stir in the salt, black pepper, and lemon juice, and remove from heat.
5. Serve immediately.

Nutrition:
Calories: 214kcal   **Fat:** 9.5   **Fiber:** 2.3g   **Carbohydrates:** 3.1g   **Protein:** 4.2 g

TEMPURA ZUCCHINI WITH CREAM CHEESE DIP

Prep Time: 15 min   **Cooking time:** 15 min   **Servings:** 4

Ingredients:

Tempura zucchinis:

- 1 1/2 cups (200 g) almond flour
- 2 tbsp. heavy cream
- 1 tsp. salt
- 2 tbsp. olive oil + extra for frying
- 1 1/4 cups (300 ml) water
- 1/2 tbsp. sugar-free maple syrup
- 2 large zucchinis, cut into 1-inch thick strips

Cream cheese dip:

- 8 oz cream cheese, room temperature
- 1/2 cup (113 g) sour cream
- 1 tsp. taco seasoning
- 1 scallion, chopped
- 1 green chili, deseeded and minced

Directions:

Tempura zucchinis:

1. In a bowl, mix the almond flour, heavy cream, salt, peanut oil, water, and maple syrup.
2. Dredge the zucchini strips in the mixture until well-coated.
3. Heat about four tablespoons of olive oil in a non-stick skillet.
4. Working in batches, use tongs to remove the zucchinis (draining extra liquid) into the oil.
5. Fry per side for 1 to 2 minutes and remove the zucchinis onto a paper towel-lined plate to drain grease.
6. Enjoy the zucchinis.

Cream cheese dip:

7. In a bowl or container, the cream cheese, taco seasoning, sour cream, scallion, and green chili must be mixed,
8. Serve the tempura zucchinis with the cream cheese dip.

Nutrition:
Calories: 316kcal   **Fat:** 8.4   **Fiber:** 9.3g   **Carbohydrates:** 4.1g   **Protein:** 5.1 g

BACON AND FETA SKEWERS

Prep Time: 15 min   **Cooking time:** 10 min   **Servings:** 4

Ingredients:

- 2 lb. feta cheese, cut into 8 cubes
- 8 bacon slices
- 4 bamboo skewers, soaked
- 1 zucchini, cut into 8 bite-size cubes
- Salt and black pepper to taste
- 3 tbsp. almond oil for brushing

Directions:

1. Wrap each feta cube with a bacon slice.
2. Thread one wrapped feta on a skewer; add a zucchini cube, then another wrapped feta, and another zucchini.
3. Repeat the threading process with the remaining skewers.
4. Preheat a grill pan to medium heat, generously brush with the avocado oil and grill the skewer on both sides for 3 to 4 minutes per side or until the set is golden brown and the bacon cooked.
5. Serve afterward with the tomato salsa.

Nutrition:
Calories: 290kcal   **Fat:** 15.1   **Fiber:** 4.2g   **Carbohydrates:** 4.1g   **Protein:** 11.8 g

AVOCADO AND PROSCIUTTO DEVILED EGGS

Prep Time: 20min **Cooking time:** 10 min **Servings:** 4

Ingredients:

- 4 eggs
- Ice bath
- 4 prosciutto slices, chopped
- 1 avocado, pitted and peeled
- 1 tbsp. mustard
- 1 tsp. plain vinegar
- 1 tbsp. heavy cream
- 1 tbsp. chopped fresh cilantro
- Salt and black pepper to taste
- 1/2 cup (113 g) mayonnaise
- 1 tbsp. coconut cream
- 1/4 tsp. cayenne pepper
- 1 tbsp. avocado oil
- 1 tbsp. chopped fresh parsley

Directions:

1. Boil the eggs for 8 minutes.
2. Remove the eggs into the ice bath, sit for 3 minutes, and then peel the eggs.
3. Slice the eggs lengthwise into halves and empty the egg yolks into a bowl.
4. Arrange the egg whites on a plate with the hole side facing upwards.
5. While the eggs are cooked, heat a non-stick skillet over medium heat and cook the prosciutto for 5 to 8 minutes.
6. Remove the prosciutto onto a paper towel-lined plate to drain grease.
7. Put the avocado slices to the egg yolks and mash both ingredients with a fork until smooth.
8. Mix in the mustard, vinegar, heavy cream, cilantro, salt, and black pepper until well-blended.
9. Spoon the mixture into a piping bag and press the mixture into the egg holes until well-filled.
10. In a bowl, whisk the mayonnaise, coconut cream, cayenne pepper, and **avocado oil.**
11. On serving plates, spoon some of the mayonnaise sauce and slightly smear it in a circular movement. Top with the deviled eggs, scatter the prosciutto on top and garnish with the parsley.
12. Enjoy immediately.

Nutrition:
Calories: 265kcal **Fat:** 11.7 **Fiber:** 4.1g **Carbohydrates:** 3.1g **Protein:** 7.9 g

CHILI-LIME TUNA SALAD

Prep Time: 10 min **Cooking time:** 0 min **Servings:** 2

Ingredients:

- 1 tablespoon of lime juice
- 1/3 cup of mayonnaise
- 1/4 teaspoon of salt
- 1 teaspoon of Tajin chili lime seasoning
- 1/8 teaspoon of pepper
- 1 medium stalk celery (finely chopped)
- 2 cups of romaine lettuce (chopped roughly)
- 2 tablespoons of red onion (finely chopped)
- optional: chopped green onion, black pepper, lemon juice
- 5 oz canned tuna

Directions:

1. Using a bowl of medium size, mix some of the ingredients such as lime, pepper, and chili-lime
2. Then, add tuna and vegetables to the pot and stir. You can serve with cucumber, celery, or a bed of greens

Nutrition:
Calories: 259kcal **Fat:** 11.3 **Fiber:** 7.4g **Carbohydrates:** 2.9g **Protein:** 12.9 g

CHICKEN CLUB LETTUCE WRAPS

Prep Time: 15min **Cooking time:** 15 min **Servings:** 1

Ingredients:

- 1 head of iceberg lettuce with the core and outer leaves removed
- 1 tbsp. of mayonnaise
- 6 slices of organic chicken or turkey breast
- Bacon (2 cooked strips, halved)
- Tomato (just 2 slices

Directions:

1. Line your working surface with a large slice of parchment paper.
2. Layer 6-8 large leaves of lettuce in the center of the paper to make a base of around 9-10 inches.
3. Spread the mayo in the center and lay with chicken or turkey, bacon, and tomato.
4. Starting with the end closest to you, roll the wrap like a jelly roll with the parchment paper as your guide. Keep it tight and halfway through, roll tuck in the ends of the wrap.
5. When it is completely wrapped, roll the rest of the parchment paper around it, and use a knife to cut it in half.

Nutrition:
Calories: 179kcal **Fat:** 4.1 **Fiber:** 9.7g **Carbohydrates:** 1.3g **Protein:** 8.5 g

CRAB-STUFFED AVOCADO

Prep Time: 20 min   **Cooking time:** 0 min   **Servings:** 2

Ingredients:

- 1 avocado, peeled, halved lengthwise, and pitted
- 1/2 teaspoon freshly squeezed lemon juice
- 41/2 ounces Dungeness crabmeat
- 1/2 cup cream cheese
- 1/4 cup chopped red bell pepper
- 1/4 cup chopped, peeled English cucumber
- 1/2 scallion, chopped
- 1 teaspoon chopped cilantro
- Pinch sea salt
- Freshly ground black pepper

Directions:

1. Brush the cut edges of the avocado with the lemon juice and set the halves aside on a plate.
2. In a bowl or container, the crabmeat, cream cheese, red pepper, cucumber, scallion, cilantro, salt, and pepper must be well mixed.
3. The crab mixture will then be divided between the avocado

Nutrition:
Calories: 239kcal   **Fat:** 11.4   **Fiber:** 8.1g   **Carbohydrates:** 3.8g   **Protein:** 5.9 g

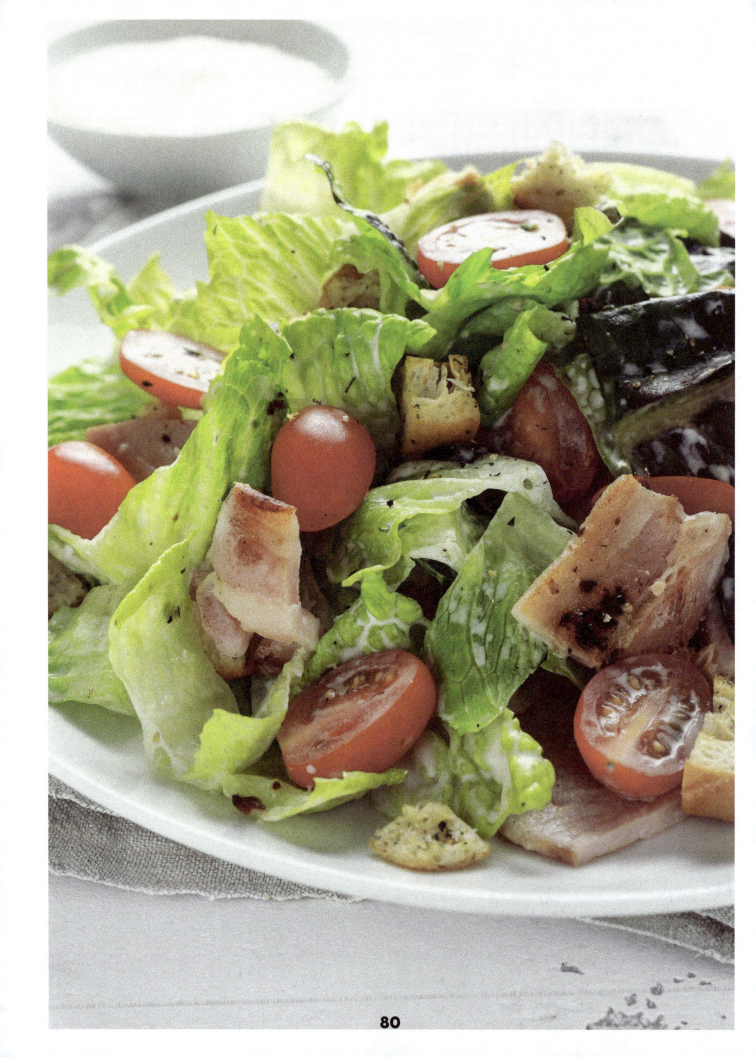

BLT SALAD

Prep Time: 15 min   **Cooking time:** 0 min   **Servings:** 4

Ingredients:

- 2 tablespoons melted bacon fat
- 2 tablespoons red wine vinegar
- Freshly ground black pepper
- 4 cups shredded lettuce
- 1 tomato, chopped
- 6 bacon slices, cooked and chopped
- 2 hardboiled eggs, chopped
- 1 tablespoon roasted unsalted sunflower seeds
- 1 teaspoon toasted sesame seeds
- 1 cooked chicken breast, sliced (optional)

Directions:

1. In a medium bowl, whisk together the bacon fat and vinegar until emulsified. Season with black pepper.
2. Add the tomato and lettuce to the bowl and toss the vegetables with the dressing.
3. Divide the salad between 4 plates and top each with equal amounts of bacon, egg, sunflower seeds, sesame seeds, and chicken (if using). Serve.

Nutrition:
Calories: 287kcal   **Fat:** 9.4   **Fiber:** 11 g   **Carbohydrates:** 3.8g   **Protein:** 9.9 g

GRILLED HALLOUMI CHEESE WITH EGGS

Prep Time: 15 min   **Cooking time:** 10 min   **Servings:** 4

Ingredients:

- 4 slices halloumi cheese
- 3 tsp. olive oil
- 1 tsp. dried Greek seasoning blend
- 1 tbsp. olive oil
- 6 eggs, beaten
- 1/2 tsp. sea salt
- 1/4 tsp. crushed red pepper flakes
- 1 1/2 cups avocado, pitted and sliced
- 1 cup grape tomatoes, halved
- 4 tbsp. pecans, chopped

Directions:

1. Preheat your grill to medium.
2. Set the Halloumi in the center of a piece of heavy-duty foil.
3. Sprinkle oil over the Halloumi and apply Greek seasoning blend.
4. Close the foil to create a packet.
5. Grill for about 15 minutes, then slice into four pieces.
6. In a frying pan, warm one tablespoon of oil and cook the eggs.
7. Stir well to create large and soft curds—season with salt and pepper.
8. Put the eggs and grilled cheese on a serving bowl.
9. Serve alongside tomatoes and avocado, decorated with chopped pecans.

Nutrition:
Calories: 219kcal   **Fat:** 5.1   **Fiber:** 4.9 g   **Carbohydrates:** 1.5g   **Protein:** 3.9 g

CREAMY KALE SALAD

Prep Time: 15 min   **Cooking time:** 0 min   **Servings:** 3

Ingredients:

- 1 bunch spinach
- 1 1/2 tablespoon lemon juice
- 1 cup sour cream
- 1 cup roasted macadamia
- 2 tablespoons sesame seeds oil
- 1 1/2 garlic clove, minced
- 1/2 teaspoon black pepper
- 1/4 teaspoon salt
- 2 tablespoons lime juice
- 1 bunch kale

Toppings:
- 1 1/2 Avocado, diced
- 1/4 cup Pecans, chopped

Directions:

1. First of all, please confirm you've all the ingredients out there. Chop kale and wash kale then remove the ribs.
2. Now transfer kale to a large bowl.
3. One thing remains to be done. Add sour cream, lime juice, macadamia, sesame seeds oil, pepper, salt, garlic.
4. Finally, mix thoroughly. Top with your avocado and pecans. Serve& enjoy.

Nutrition:
Calories: 291kcal   **Fat:** 5.1   **Fiber:** 12.9g   **Carbohydrates:** 4.3g   **Protein:** 11.8 g

QUINOA SALAD WITH FRESH MINT AND PARSLEY

 Prep Time: 10 min   **Cooking time:** 15 min **Servings:** 4

Ingredients:

- 2 cups of quinoa
- 1/2 cup of almond nut
- 3 tablespoons of fresh parsley (chopped)
- 1/2 cup of chopped green onions
- 3 tablespoons of chopped fresh mint
- 3 tablespoons of olive oil
- 2 tablespoons of lemon juice
- 1 teaspoon of garlic salt
- 1/2 teaspoon of salt and pepper

Directions:

1. Place a saucepan on high heat.
2. Add the quinoa and water and just let it boil for around 15 minutes, then reduce the heat and drain.
3. Pour the drained quinoa in a large bowl, add the parsley, almond nuts, and mint.
4. In a bowl or container, add the olive oil, garlic salt, and lemon juice together.
5. Whisk the mixture well until it's well combined and pour over the quinoa.
6. Combine the mixture well until everything is well dispersed.
7. Add the salt and black pepper to taste.
8. Place the quinoa mixture bowl in the refrigerator.

Nutrition:
Calories: 241kcal   **Fat:** 8.4   **Fiber:** 11.4 g   **Carbohydrates:** 2.1 g   **Protein:** 9.3 g

BRUSSEL SPROUTS WITH BACON

Prep Time: 5 min **Cooking time:** 40 min **Servings:** 6

Ingredients:

- 16 ounces Brussel sprouts
- 1 teaspoon salt
- 16 ounces bacon, pasteurized
- 2/3 teaspoon ground black pepper

Directions:

1. Preheat oven to 400°F.
2. Slice every sprout in half and then slice bacon lengthwise into small pieces.
3. Take a baking sheet, line it with parchment paper, spread Brussel sprouts halves and bacon on it, and then season with salt and black pepper.
4. Bake for 35–40 minutes until sprouts turn golden-brown, and bacon is crisp.
5. Serve straight away.

Nutrition:
Calories: 101kcal **Fat:** 5.1 g **Fiber:** 10 g **Carbohydrates:** 1 g **Protein:** 5.5 g

SMOKED SALMON AND CREAM CHEESE ROLL-UPS

Prep Time: 25 min

Cooking time: 0 min

Servings: 2

Ingredients:

- 4 ounces cream cheese, at room temperature
- 1 teaspoon grated lemon zest
- 1 teaspoon Dijon mustard
- 2 tablespoons chopped scallions
- Pink Himalayan salt
- Freshly ground black pepper
- 1 package cold-smoked salmon

Directions:

1. Put the cream cheese, lemon zest, mustard, scallions in a food processor (or blender), and season with pink Himalayan salt and pepper.
2. Process until thoroughly mixed and smooth.
3. Spread the cream cheese on each pc. of smoked salmon, and roll it up.
4. Place the rolls on a plate seam-side down.
5. Serve immediately or refrigerate.

Nutrition:
Calories: 334kcal **Fat:** 12.6 **Fiber:** 3.1g **Carbohydrates:** 2.2g **Protein:** 15.1 g

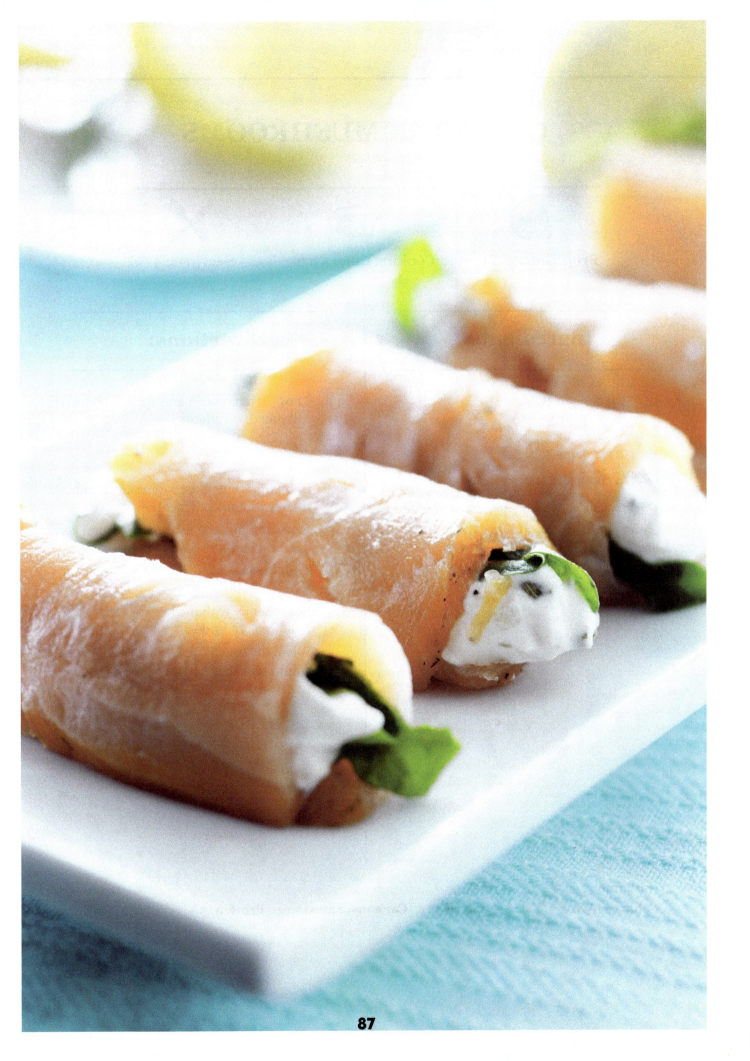

CRABMEAT MUSHROOMS

Prep Time: 5 min   **Cooking time:** 5 min   **Servings:** 4

Ingredients:

- 7 oz. crab meat
- 10 oz. white mushrooms
- 1/2 teaspoon salt
- 1/4 cup fish stock
- 1 teaspoon butter
- 1/4 teaspoon ground coriander
- 1 teaspoon dried cilantro
- 1 teaspoon butter

Directions:

1. Chop the crab meat and sprinkle it with the salt and dried cilantro.
2. Mix the crab meat carefully.
3. Preheat the air fryer to 400 F.
4. Chop the white mushrooms and combine them with the crab meat.
5. After this, add the fish stock, ground coriander, and butter.
6. Transfer the side dish mixture in the air fryer basket tray.
7. Stir it gently with the help of the plastic spatula. Cook the side dish for 5 minutes.
8. When the time is over – let the dish rest for 5 minutes. Then serve it. Enjoy!

Nutrition:
Calories: 198kcal   **Fat:** 8 g   **Fiber:** 3.1g   **Carbohydrates:** 1.2g   **Protein:** 5.5 g

GRILLED MEDITERRANEAN VEGGIES

Prep Time: 10 min   **Cooking time:** 15 min   **Servings:** 4

Ingredients:

- 1/4 cup (56 g/2 oz) ghee or butter
- 2 small (200 g/7.1 oz) red, orange, or yellow peppers
- 3 medium (600 g/21.2 oz) zucchini
- 1 medium (500 g/17.6 oz) eggplant
- 1 medium (100 g/3.5 oz) red onion

Directions:

1. Set the oven to broil to the highest setting.
2. In a small bowl, mix the melted ghee and crushed garlic.
3. Wash all the vegetables.
4. Halve, deseed, and slice the bell peppers into strips.
5. Slice the zucchini widthwise into 1/4-inch (about 1/2 cm) pieces.
6. Wash the eggplant and slice.
7. Quarter each slice into 1/4-inch (about 1/2 cm) pieces.
8. Peel and slice the onion into medium wedges and separate the sections using your hands.
9. Place the vegetables in a bowl and add the chopped herbs, ghee with garlic, salt, and black pepper. The vegetables must be spread on a baking sheet, ideally on a roasting rack or net, so that the vegetables don't become soggy from the juices.
10. Put it in the oven and let it cook for about 15 minutes.
11. Be careful not to burn them.
12. When done, the vegetables should be slightly tender but still crisp.
13. Serve with meat dishes or bake with cheese such as feta, mozzarella, or Halloumi.

Nutrition:
Calories: 176kcal   **Fat:** 4.5 g   **Fiber:** 9.3 g   **Carbohydrates:** 3.1 g   **Protein:** 5.2 g

BACON AND WILD MUSHROOMS

Prep Time: 10 min

Cooking time: 15 min

Servings: 4

Ingredients:

- 6 strips uncured bacon, chopped
- 4 cups sliced wild mushrooms
- 2 teaspoons minced garlic
- 2 tablespoons chicken stock
- 1 tablespoon chopped fresh thyme

Directions:

1. Cook the bacon. In a pot, cook the bacon until it's crispy and cooked through, about 7 minutes.
2. Cook the mushrooms. Add the mushrooms and garlic and sauté until the mushrooms are tender about 7 minutes.
3. Deglaze the pan. Add the chicken stock and stir to scrape up any browned bits in the bottom of the pan.
4. Garnish and serve. Put the mushrooms in a bowl, sprinkle them with the thyme, and serve.

Nutrition:
Calories: 175kcal **Fat:** 4.9 g **Fiber:** 8.4 g **Carbohydrates:** 2.2g **Protein:** 1.4 g

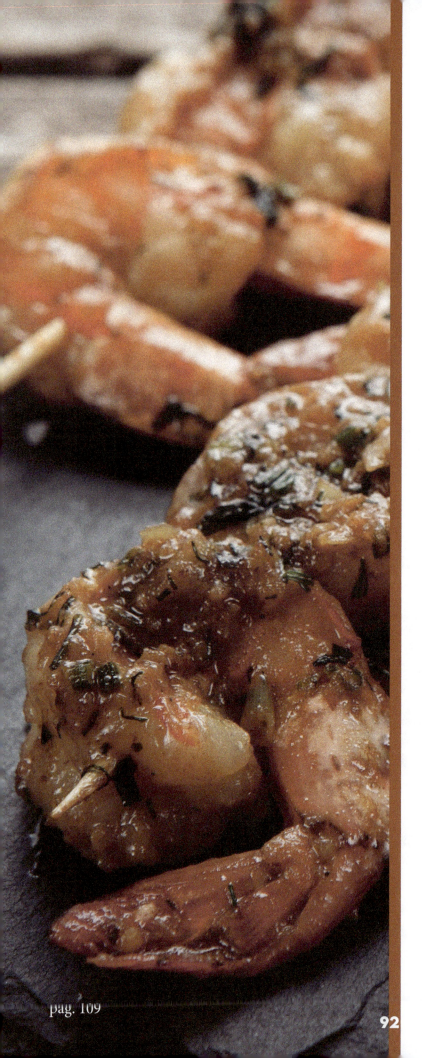

12

SEAFOODS RECIPES

LEMONY SEA BASS FILLET

 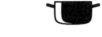

Prep Time: 10 min   **Cooking time:** 15 min   **Servings:** 4

Ingredients:

Fish:

- 4 sea bass fillets
- 2 tablespoons olive oil, divided
- A pinch of chili pepper
- Salt, to taste

Olive Sauce:

- 1 tablespoon green olives, pitted and sliced
- 1 lemon, juiced
- Salt, to taste

Directions:

1. Preheat the grill to high heat.
2. Stir together one tablespoon olive oil, chili pepper, and salt in a bowl.
3. Brush both sides of each sea bass fillet generously with the mixture.
4. Grill the fillets on the preheated grill for about 5 to 6 minutes on each side until lightly browned.
5. Meanwhile, warm the left olive oil in a skillet over medium heat.
6. Add the green olives, lemon juice, and salt.
7. Cook until the sauce is heated through.
8. Transfer the fillets to four serving plates, then pour the sauce over them. Serve warm.

Nutrition:
Calories: 257kcal   **Fat:** 12.4 g   **Fiber:** 5.6 g   **Carbohydrates:** 2g   **Protein:** 12.7 g

CURRIED FISH WITH SUPER GREENS

Prep Time: 10 min   **Cooking time:** 20 min   **Servings:** 4

Ingredients:

- 2 tablespoons coconut oil
- 2 teaspoons garlic, minced
- 1 1/2 tablespoons grated fresh ginger
- 1/2 teaspoon ground cumin
- 1 tablespoon curry powder
- 2 cups of coconut milk
- 16 ounces (454 g) firm white fish, cut into 1-inch chunks
- 1 cup kale, shredded
- 2 tablespoons cilantro, chopped

Directions:

1. Melt the coconut oil in a heated pan
2. Add the garlic and ginger and sauté for about 2 minutes until tender.
3. Fold in the cumin and curry powder, then cook for 1 to 2 minutes until fragrant.
4. Put in the coconut milk and boil. Boil then simmer until the flavors mellow, about 5 minutes.
5. Add the fish chunks and simmer for 10 minutes until the fish flakes easily with a fork, stirring once.
6. Scatter the shredded kale and chopped cilantro over the fish, then cook for 2 minutes more until softened.

Nutrition:
Calories: 376kcal   **Fat:** 19.9 g   **Fiber:** 15.8 g   **Carbohydrates:** 6.7g   **Protein:** 14.8 g

SHRIMP ALFREDO

Prep Time: 15 min   **Cooking time:** 30 min   **Servings:** 4

Ingredients:

- 1 pound of wild shrimp
- 3 tablespoons of organic grass-fed whey
- 1 1/2 cups of frozen asparagus
- 1 cup of heavy cream
- 1/2 cup of parmesan cheese
- Sea salt
- Black pepper
- 2 ground garlic cloves
- 1 small diced onion

Directions:

1. Peel and devein the shrimps, coat them well with salt and pepper. Let it cover in a bowl for 20 minutes.
2. Preheat a skillet. Put in butter, garlic, and onions.
3. When butter is melted, put in shrimp and stir fry till for 3 minutes.
4. Pour in heavy cream and stir well. Then, add ion cheese and stir till cheese melts.
5. Serve hot

Nutrition:
Calories: 315kcal   **Fat:** 11.9 g   **Fiber:** 8.5 g   **Carbohydrates:** 9.3 g   **Protein:** 11.1 g

GARLIC-LEMON MAHI MAHI

Prep Time: 15 min   **Cooking time:** 10 min   **Servings:** 3

Ingredients:

- 6 tablespoons of butter
- 5 tablespoons of extra-virgin olive oil
- 4 ounces of mahi-mahi fillets
- 3 minced cloves of garlic
- Kosher salt
- Black pepper
- 2 pounds of asparagus
- 2 sliced lemons
- Zest and juice of 2 lemons
- 1 teaspoon of crushed red pepper flakes
- 1 tablespoon of chopped parsley

Directions:

1. Melt three tablespoons of butter and olive oil in a microwave.
2. Heat a skillet and put in mahi-mahi, then sprinkle black pepper.
3. For around 5 minutes per side, cook it. When done, move to a plate.
4. In another skillet, add remaining oil and add in the asparagus, stir fry for 2-3 minutes. Take out on a plate.
5. In the same skillet, pour in the remaining butter, and add garlic, red pepper, lemon, zest, juice, and parsley.
6. Add in the mahi-mahi and asparagus and stir together. Serve hot.

Nutrition:
Calories: 317kcal   **Fat:** 8.5 g   **Fiber:** 6.9 g   **Carbohydrates:** 3.1g   **Protein:** 16.1 g

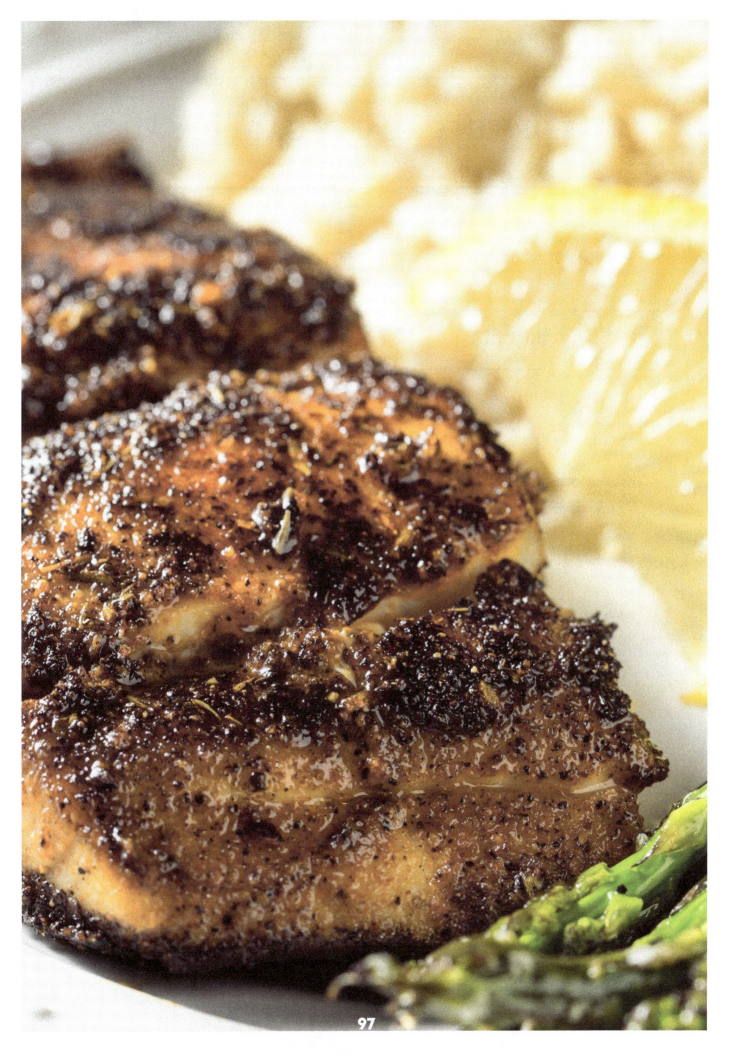

SCALLOPS IN CREAMY GARLIC SAUCE

Prep Time: 15 min   **Cooking time:** 15 min   **Servings:** 4

Ingredients:

- 11/4 pounds fresh sea scallops, side muscles removed
- Salt and ground black pepper, as required
- 4 tablespoons butter, divided
- 5 garlic cloves, chopped
- 1/4 cup homemade chicken broth
- 1 cup heavy cream
- 1 tablespoon fresh lemon juice
- 2 tablespoons fresh parsley, chopped

Directions:

1. Sprinkle the scallops evenly with salt and black pepper.
2. Melt two tablespoons of butter in a large pan over medium-high heat and cook the scallops for about 2–3 minutes per side.
3. Flip the scallops and cook for about two more minutes.
4. With a slotted spoon, transfer the scallops onto a plate.
5. Using the same pan, the butter must be melted and sauté the garlic for about 1 minute.
6. Pour the broth and bring to a gentle boil.
7. Cook for about 2 minutes.
8. Stir in the cream and cook for about 1–2 minutes or until slightly thickened.
9. Stir in the cooked scallops and lemon juice and remove from heat.
10. Garnish with fresh parsley and serve hot.

Nutrition:
Calories: 259kcal   **Fat:** 8.5 g   **Fiber:** 7.4 g   **Carbohydrates:** 2.1 g   **Protein:** 12.2 g

SHRIMP CURRY

Prep Time: 15 min   **Cooking time:** 20 min   **Servings:** 4

Ingredients:

- 2 tablespoons coconut oil
- 1/2 of yellow onion, minced
- 2 garlic cloves, minced
- 1 teaspoon ground turmeric
- 1 teaspoon ground cumin
- 1 teaspoon paprika
- 1 (14-ounce) can unsweetened coconut milk
- 1 large tomato, chopped finely
- Salt, as required
- 1-pound shrimp, peeled and deveined
- 2 tablespoons fresh cilantro, chopped

Directions:

1. The coconut oil must be melted in a wok medium heat and sauté the onion for about 5 minutes.
2. Add the garlic and spices, and sauté for about 1 minute.
3. Add the coconut milk, tomato, and salt, and bring to a gentle boil.
4. Let the curry simmer for about 10 minutes, stirring occasionally.
5. Stir in the shrimp and cilantro and simmer for about 4–5 minutes.

Nutrition:
Calories: 354kcal   **Fat:** 12.5 g   **Fiber:** 7.5 g   **Carbohydrates:** 4.1g   **Protein:** 14.1 g

ISRAELI SALMON SALAD

Prep Time: 10 min   **Cooking time:** 0 min   **Servings:** 2

Ingredients:

- 1 cup flaked smoked salmon
- 1 tomato, chopped
- 1/2 small red onion, chopped
- 1 cucumber, chopped
- 6 tbsp. pitted green olives
- 1 avocado, chopped
- 2 tbsp. avocado oil
- 2 tbsp. almond oil
- 1 tbsp. plain vinegar
- Salt and black pepper to taste
- 1 cup crumbled feta cheese
- 1 cup grated cheddar cheese

Directions:

1. In a salad bowl, add the salmon, tomatoes, red onion, cucumber, green olives, and avocado. Mix well.
2. In a bowl, whisk the avocado oil, vinegar, salt, and black pepper.
3. Drizzle the dressing over the salad and toss well.
4. Sprinkle some feta cheese and serve the salad immediately.

Nutrition:
Calories: 415kcal   **Fat:** 11.4 g   **Fiber:** 9.9 g   **Carbohydrates:** 3.8 g   **Protein:** 15.4 g

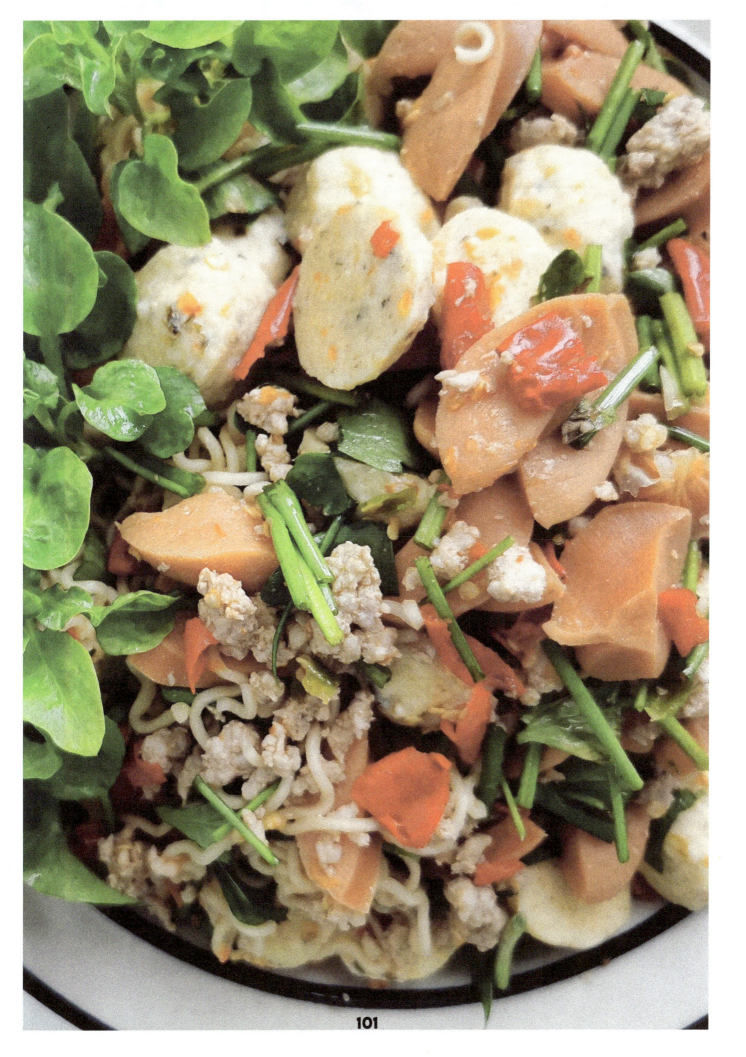

GREEK TUNA SALAD

Prep Time: 10 min **Cooking time:** 0 min **Servings:** 2

Ingredients:

- 3 cans tuna
- 1/4 small red onion, finely chopped
- 1 celery stalks, finely chopped
- 1/2 avocado, chopped
- 1 tbsp. chopped fresh parsley
- 1 cup Greek yogurt
- 2 tbsp. butter
- 2 tsp. Dijon Mustard
- 1/2 tbsp. vinegar
- Salt and black pepper to taste

Directions:

1. The ingredients listed must be added to a salad bowl and mix until well combined.
2. Serve afterward.

Nutrition:
Calories: 376kcal **Fat:** 10.4 g **Fiber:** 11.9 g **Carbohydrates:** 3.9g **Protein:** 18.4 g

BLACKENED SALMON WITH AVOCADO SALSA

Prep Time: 15 min   **Cooking time:** 10 min   **Servings:** 4

Ingredients:

- 1 tbsp. extra virgin olive oil
- 4 filets of salmon (about 6 oz. each)
- 4 tsp. Cajun seasoning
- 2 med. avocados, diced
- 1 c. cucumber, diced
- 1/4 c. red onion, diced
- 1 tbsp. parsley, chopped
- 1 tbsp. lime juice
- Sea salt & pepper, to taste

Directions:

1. The oil must be heated in a skillet.
2. Rub the Cajun seasoning into the fillets, then lay them into the bottom of the skillet once it's hot enough.
3. Cook until a dark crust forms, then flip and repeat.
4. In a medium mixing bowl, combine all the ingredients for the salsa and set aside.
5. Plate the fillets and top with 1/4 of the salsa yielded.
6. Enjoy!

Nutrition:
Calories: 425kcal   **Fat:** 15.8 g   **Fiber:** 19.2 g   **Carbohydrates:** 4.1 g   **Protein:** 11.8 g

TANGY COCONUT COD

 Prep Time: 10 min   **Cooking time:** 10 min   **Servings:** 2

Ingredients:

- 1/3 c. coconut flour
- 1/2 tsp. cayenne pepper
- 1 egg, beaten
- 1 lime
- 1 tsp. crushed red pepper flakes
- 1 tsp. garlic powder
- 12 oz. cod fillets
- Sea salt & pepper, to taste

Directions:

1. Let the oven preheat to 400°F/175°C. then line a baking sheet with non-stick foil.
2. Place the flour in a shallow dish (a plate works fine) and drag the fillets of cod through the beaten egg. Dredge the cod in the coconut flour, then lay on the baking sheet.
3. Sprinkle the fillet's top with the seasoning and lime juice.
4. Bake the cod for about 10 to 12 minutes until the fillets are flaky.
5. Serve immediately!

Nutrition:
Calories: 318kcal   **Fat:** 12.1 g   **Fiber:** 15.1 g   **Carbohydrates:** 4.1 g   **Protein:** 19.5 g

FISH TACO BOWL

Prep Time: 10 min **Cooking time:** 15 min **Servings:** 2

Ingredients:

- 2 (5-ounce) tilapia fillets
- 1 tablespoon olive oil
- 4 teaspoons Tajin seasoning salt, divided
- 2 cups pre-sliced coleslaw cabbage mix
- 1 tablespoon avocado mayo
- 1 tsp. hot sauce
- 1 avocado, mashed
- Pink Himalayan salt
- Freshly ground black pepper

Directions:

1. Preheat the oven to 425°F. The baking sheet must be lined with a baking mat.
2. Rub the tilapia with the olive oil, and then coat it with two teaspoons of Tajín seasoning salt.
3. Place the fish in the prepared pan.
4. Let the tilapia bake for 15 minutes, or until the fish is opaque when you pierce it with a fork.
5. Meanwhile, in a medium bowl, gently mix to combine the coleslaw and the mayo sauce.
6. You don't want the cabbage super wet, just enough to dress it.
7. Add the mashed avocado and the remaining two teaspoons of Tajín seasoning salt to the coleslaw, and season with pink Himalayan salt and pepper.
8. Divide the salad between two bowls.
9. Shred fish into tiny pieces, and add it to the bowls.
10. Top the fish with a drizzle of mayo sauce and serve.

Nutrition:
Calories: 231kcal **Fat:** 12.1 g **Fiber:** 10.3 g **Carbohydrates:** 2.1 g **Protein:** 17.3 g

SCALLOPS WITH CREAMY BACON SAUCE

Prep Time: 5 min   **Cooking time:** 20 min   **Servings:** 2

Ingredients:

- 4 bacon slices
- 1 cup heavy (whipping) cream
- 1 tablespoon butter
- 1/4 cup grated Parmesan cheese
- Pink Himalayan salt
- Freshly ground black pepper
- 1 tablespoon ghee
- 8 large sea scallops, rinsed and patted dry

Directions:

1. Cook the bacon.
2. Lower the heat to medium. Add the butter, cream, and Parmesan cheese to the bacon grease and season with a pinch of pink Himalayan salt and pepper.
3. Lower the heat down, then stir constantly until the sauce thickens and is reduced by 50 percent, about 10 minutes.
4. In another skillet, heat the ghee until sizzling.
5. Season the scallops with pink Himalayan salt and pepper, and add them to the skillet—Cook for just 1 minute per side.
6. Do not crowd the scallops; if your pan isn't large enough, cook them in two batches.
7. You want the scallops golden on each side.
8. Transfer the scallops to a paper towel-lined plate.
9. Divide the cream sauce between two plates, crumble the bacon on top of the cream sauce, and top with four scallops. Serve immediately.

Nutrition:
Calories: 311kcal   **Fat:** 14.1 g   **Fiber:** 10.3 g   **Carbohydrates:** 1.2 g   **Protein:** 17.7 g

PARMESAN-GARLIC SALMON WITH ASPARAGUS

Prep Time: 10 min   **Cooking time:** 15 min   **Servings:** 2

Ingredients:

- 2 (6-ounce) salmon fillets, skin on
- Pink Himalayan salt
- Freshly ground black pepper
- 1-pound fresh asparagus ends snapped off
- 3 tablespoons butter
- 2 garlic cloves, minced
- 1/4 cup grated Parmesan cheese

Directions:

1. Oven: 400°F.
2. Pat the salmon dry and season both sides with pink Himalayan salt and pepper.
3. Put the salmon, and arrange the asparagus around the salmon.
4. Melt the butter. Add the minced garlic and stir until the garlic just begins to brown about 3 minutes.
5. Drizzle the garlic-butter sauce over the salmon and asparagus, and top both with the Parmesan cheese.
6. Bake until the salmon is cooked and the asparagus is crisp-tender, about 12 minutes. You can switch the oven to broil at the end of cooking time to char the asparagus.
7. Serve hot.

Nutrition:
Calories: 476 kcal   **Fat:** 14.1 g   **Fiber:** 10.5 g   **Carbohydrates:** 3.1 g   **Protein:** 19.9 g

SPICY SHRIMP SKEWERS

Prep Time: 5 min   **Cooking time:** 3/9 min   **Servings:** 4

Ingredients:

- 2 tbsp. Paprika
- 1/2 tbsp. Onion powder
- 1/2 tbsp. dried thyme, crushed
- 1-pound shrimp, peeled and deveined
- 2 tbsp. Olive oil
- 1/2 tbsp. Red chili powder
- 1/2 tbsp. Garlic powder
- 1/2 tbsp. dried oregano, crushed
- 2 zucchinis, cut into 1/2-inch cubes

Directions:

1. Preheat the grill to medium-high heat.
2. In a bowl, mix spices and dried herbs.
3. In a large bowl, add shrimp, zucchini, oil, and seasoning and toss to coat well.
4. Thread shrimp and zucchini onto pre-soaked skewers.
5. Grill the skewers for about 6-8 minutes, flipping occasionally. Serve hot.

Nutrition:
Calories: 261 kcal   **Fat:** 9.4 g   **Fiber:** 10.1 g   **Carbohydrates:** 3.2 g   **Protein:** 4.1 g

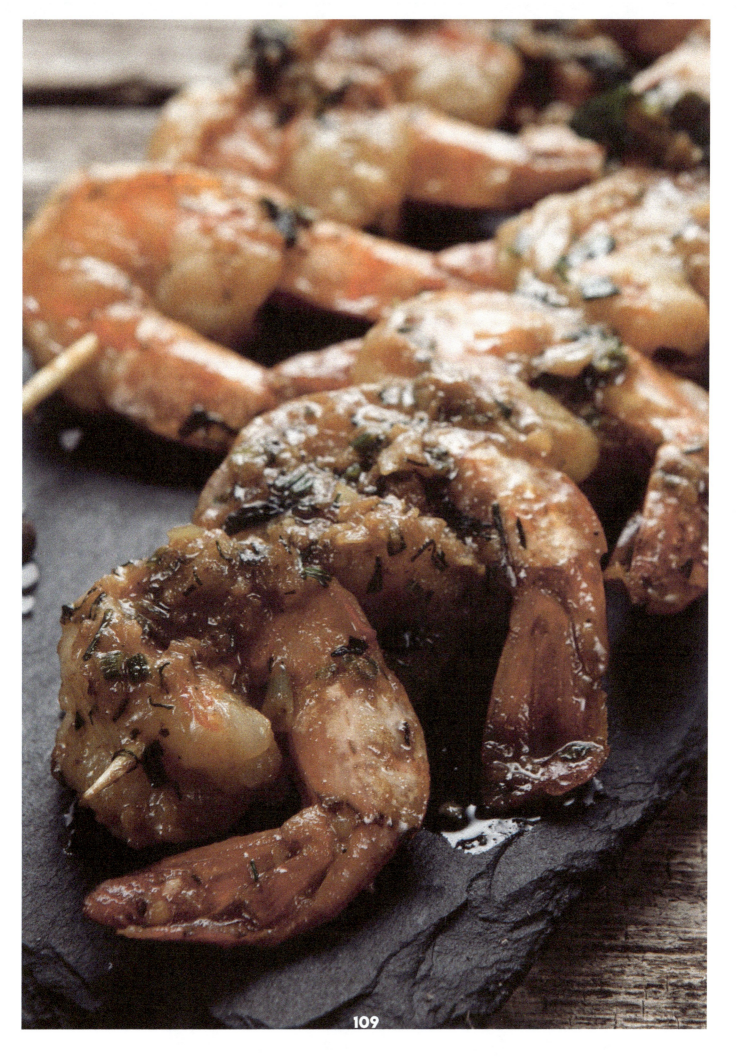

FRIED SHRIMP TAILS

 Prep Time: 10 min    **Cooking time:** 15 min   **Servings:** 4

Ingredients:

- 1-pound shrimp tails
- 1 tablespoon olive oil
- 1 teaspoon dried dill
- 1/2 teaspoon dried parsley
- 2 tablespoon coconut flour
- 1/2 cup heavy cream
- 1 teaspoon chili flakes

Directions:

1. Peel the shrimp tails and sprinkle them with the dried dill and dried parsley.
2. Mix the shrimp tails carefully in the mixing bowl.
3. After this, combine the coconut flour, heavy cream, and chili flakes in the separate bowl and whisk it until you get the smooth batter.
4. Then preheat the air fryer to 330 F.
5. Transfer the shrimp tails in the heavy crema batter and stir the seafood carefully.
6. Then spray the air fryer rack and put the shrimp tails there.
7. Cook the shrimp tails for 7 minutes. After this, turn the shrimp tails into another side.
8. Cook the shrimp tails for 7 minutes more. When the seafood is cooked – chill it well. Enjoy!

Nutrition:
Calories: 212 kcal   **Fat:** 10.1 g   **Fiber:** 8.5 g   **Carbohydrates:** 2.6 g   **Protein:** 5.1 g

CAJUN LOBSTER TAILS

 Prep Time: 10 min

 Cooking time: 20 min

 Servings: 4

Ingredients:

- 1 lb. of peeled and deveined raw Lobster
- 1 Cup of almond flour
- 1 tbsp. of pepper
- 1 tbsp. of salt
- 1 tsp. of cayenne pepper
- 1 tsp. of cumin
- 1 tsp. of garlic powder
- 1 tbsp. of paprika
- 1 tbsp. of onion powder

Directions:

1. Preheat your fryer to a temperature of 390° F. Peel the lobster and devein it.
2. Dip in the lobster into the heavy cream.
3. Dredge the lobster into the mixture of the almond flour. Shake off any excess of flour.
4. Put the lobster in the fryer and cook for about 15 minutes and the temperature to 200° C/400° F.
5. You can check your appetizer after about 6 minutes, and you can flip the lobster if needed. Serve and enjoy your lobsters!

Nutrition:
Calories: 321 kcal **Fat:** 14.1 g **Fiber:** 12.1 g **Carbohydrates:** 3.2 g **Protein:** 8.5 g

KETO CRISPY GINGER MACKEREL LUNCH BOWL

Prep Time: 12 min   **Cooking time:** 20 min   **Servings:** 2

Ingredients:

Marinade:

- 1 tbsp. grated ginger
- 1 tbsp. lemon juice
- 3 tbsp. olive oil
- 1 tbsp. coconut aminos
- Salt and pepper, to taste

Lunch bowl:

- 2 (8-ounce) boneless mackerel fillets
- 1-ounce almonds
- 1 1/2 cups broccoli
- 1 tbsp. butter
- 1/2 small yellow onion
- 1/3 cup diced red bell pepper
- 2 small sun-dried tomatoes, chopped
- 4 tbsp. mashed avocado

Directions:

1. Oven: 400 °F.
2. Mix the grated ginger, lemon juice, olive oil, coconut aminos, and salt and pepper.
3. Then Rub half of the marinade on the fish fillets.
4. Place the fillets onto the baking tray with the skin side facing up.
5. Roast the fish fillet for 12-15 minutes or until the skin is crispy and golden browned.
6. Almonds must be spread in an even layer and roast it until golden for 5-8 minutes.
7. Boil the broccoli until tender.
8. Melt butter.
9. Add the onions and peppers to the pan and cook until they are soft.
10. Stir in the sundried tomatoes, and just cook until warm through.
11. Stir in the rest of the dressing and top with chopped almonds.
12. Serve with the avocado.

Nutrition:
Calories: 241 kcal   **Fat:** 15.1 g   **Fiber:** 9.4 g   **Carbohydrates:** 4.1 g   **Protein:** 19.1 g

CREAMY SHRIMP SALAD

Prep Time: 10 min **Cooking time:** 5 min **Servings:** 1

Ingredients:

- 6 leaves Boston lettuce
- 10.5 oz (300g) peeled shrimp
- 1 1/2 tbsp.. olive oil
- 1/2 cup (50g) chopped celery
- 1 stalk chopped green onion
- Dressing
- 4 tbsp. mayonnaise
- 1 tbsp. heavy whipping cream
- 1/2 tsp. dill
- 1/2 tsp. dried parsley
- 1/4 tsp. paprika
- 1 tsp. lemon juice

Directions:

1. In a preheated pan, add oil
2. Put the shrimp and sauté for about 3-5 minutes or until cooked through.
3. In a salad bowl, whisk the parsley, paprika, mayonnaise, cream, dill, and lemon juice together.
4. Put the cooked shrimp to the salad bowl along with the celery and green onions.
5. Combine the shrimp and vegetables until thoroughly coat with the dressing.

Nutrition:
Calories: 376 kcal **Fat:** 14.2 g **Fiber:** 8.5 g **Carbohydrates:** 3.8 g **Protein:** 15.1 g

PAN-SEARED COD WITH TOMATO HOLLANDAISE

Prep Time: 10 min   **Cooking time:** 10 min   **Servings:** 4

Ingredients:

- Pan-Seared Cod
- 1 pound (4-fillets) wild Alaskan Cod
- 1 tbsp. salted butter
- 1 tbsp. olive oil
- Tomato Hollandaise
- 3 large egg yolks
- 3 tbsp. warm water
- 226 grams salted butter, melted
- 1/4 tsp. salt
- 1/4 tsp. black pepper
- 2 tbsp. tomato paste
- 2 tbsp. fresh lemon juice

Directions:

1. Season both sides of the code fillet without salt, the salt will be added in the last.
2. Heat a skillet over medium heat and coat with olive oil and butter.
3. When the butter heats up, place the cod fillet in the skillet and sear on both sides for 2-3 minutes. Baste the fish fillet with the oil and butter mixture.
4. You will know that the cod cooked when it easily flakes when poked with a fork.
5. Melt the butter in the microwave.
6. In a double boil, beat egg yolks with warm water until thick and creamy and start forming soft peaks. Remove the double boil from the heat, gradually adding the melted butter and stirring.
7. Season.
8. Mix in the tomato paste. Stir to combine. Pour in the water and lemon juice to lighten the sauce texture.

Nutrition:
Calories: 356 kcal   **Fat:** 16.1 g   **Fiber:** 12.3 g   **Carbohydrates:** 3.1 g   **Protein:** 18.4 g

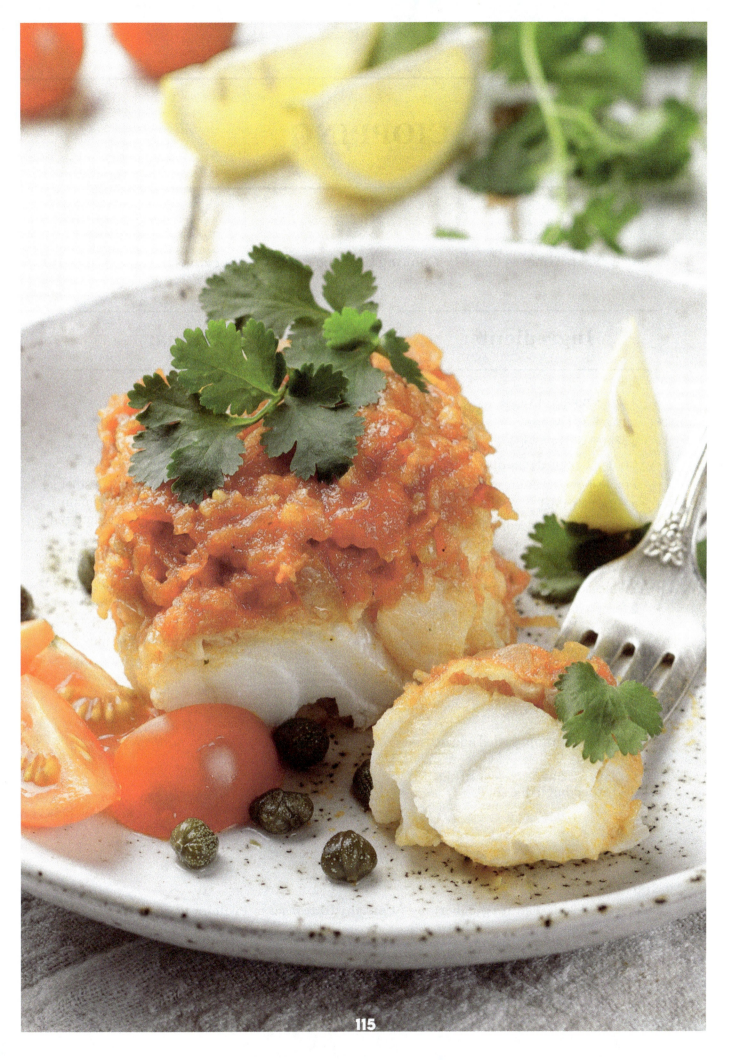

CIOPPINO

 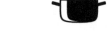

Prep Time: 15 min   **Cooking time:** 30 min   **Servings:** 6

Ingredients:

- 2 tablespoons olive oil
- 1/2 onion, chopped
- 2 celery stalks, sliced
- 1 red bell pepper, chopped
- 1 tablespoon minced garlic
- 2 cups fish stock
- 1 (15-ounce) can coconut milk
- 1 cup crushed tomatoes
- 2 tablespoons tomato paste
- 1 tablespoon chopped fresh basil
- 2 teaspoons chopped fresh oregano
- 1/2 teaspoon of sea salt
- 1/2 teaspoon freshly ground black pepper
- 1/4 teaspoon red pepper flakes
- 10 ounces salmon, cut into 1-inch pieces
- 1/2 pound shrimp, peeled and deveined
- 12 clams or mussels, cleaned and debearded but in the shell

Directions:

1. Sauté the vegetables.
2. In a pot, warm the olive oil. Add the onion, celery, red bell pepper, and garlic and sauté until they've softened about 4 minutes.
3. Make the soup base. Stir in the fish stock, coconut milk, crushed tomatoes, tomato paste, basil, oregano, salt, pepper, and red pepper flakes.
4. Boil then simmer the soup for 10 minutes.
5. Add the seafood. Stir in the salmon and simmer until it goes opaque about 5 minutes.
6. Add the shrimp and simmer until they're almost cooked through about 3 minutes. Add the mussels.
7. Serve.

Nutrition:
Calories: 321 kcal   **Fat:** 11.1 g   **Fiber:** 16 g   **Carbohydrates:** 4.2 g   **Protein:** 16.4 g

COCONUT MUSSELS

Prep Time: 10 min   **Cooking time:** 15 min   **Servings:** 4

Ingredients:

- 2 tablespoons coconut oil
- 1/2 sweet onion, chopped
- 2 teaspoons minced garlic
- 1 teaspoon grated fresh ginger
- 1/2 teaspoon turmeric
- 1 cup of coconut milk
- Juice of 1 lime
- 11/2 pounds fresh mussels, scrubbed and debearded
- 1 scallion, finely chopped
- 2 tablespoons chopped fresh cilantro
- 1 tablespoon chopped fresh thyme

Directions:

1. Sauté the aromatics.
2. In a pot, warm the coconut oil. Add the onion, garlic, ginger, and turmeric and sauté until they've softened about 3 minutes.
3. Add the liquid. Stir in the coconut milk and lime juice and bring the mixture to a boil.
4. Steam the mussels.
5. Add the mussels to the skillet, cover, and steam until the shells are open, about 10 minutes.
6. Take the skillet off the heat and throw out any unopened mussels.
7. Add the herbs. Stir in the scallion, cilantro, and thyme.
8. Serve. Divide the mussels and the sauce between four bowls and serve them immediately.

Nutrition:
Calories: 321 kcal   **Fat:** 11.1 g   **Fiber:** 9 g   **Carbohydrates:** 1.2 g   **Protein:** 1.4 g

ITALIAN STYLE HALIBUT PACKETS

 Prep Time: 10 min
 Cooking time: 20 min
 Servings: 4

Ingredients:

- 2 cups cauliflower florets
- 1 cup roasted red pepper strips
- 1/2 cup sliced sun-dried tomatoes
- 4 (4-ounce) halibut fillets
- 1/4 cup chopped fresh basil
- Juice of 1 lemon
- 1/4 cup good-quality olive oil
- Sea salt, for seasoning
- Freshly ground black pepper, for seasoning

Directions:

1. Preheat the oven. Set the oven temperature to 400°F.
2. Make the packets.
3. Divide the cauliflower, red pepper strips, and sun-dried tomato between the four pieces of foil, placing the vegetables in the middle of each piece.
4. Top each pile with one halibut fillet, and top each fillet with equal amounts of the basil, lemon juice, and olive oil.
5. Fold and crimp the foil to form sealed packets of fish and vegetables and place them on the baking sheet.
6. Bake. Bake the packets for about 20 minutes, until the fish flakes with a fork.
7. Be careful of the steam when you open the packet!
8. Serve. Transfer the vegetables and halibut to four plates, season with salt and pepper, and serve immediately.

Nutrition:
Calories: 313 kcal   **Fat:** 14.1 g   **Fiber:** 10.4 g   **Carbohydrates:** 3.2 g   **Protein:** 15.4 g

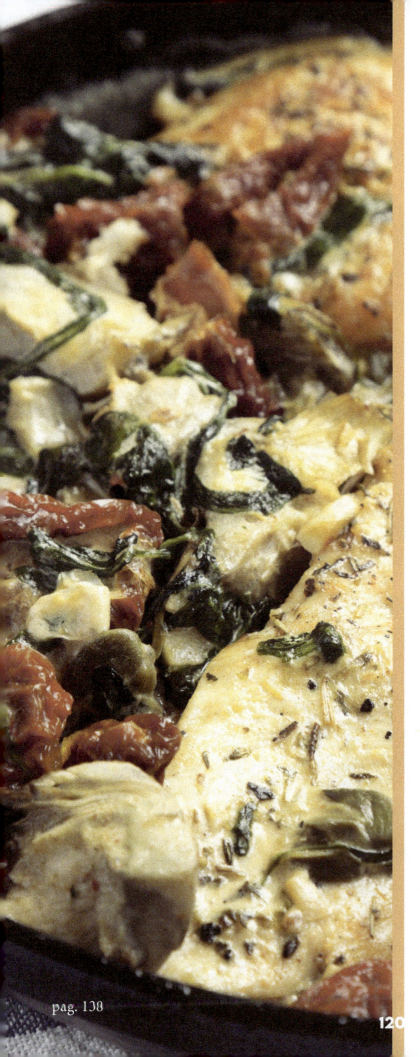

pag. 138

13

POULTRY RECIPES

CHEESY ROASTED CHICKEN

Prep Time: 15 min   **Cooking time:** 10 min   **Servings:** 6

Ingredients:

- 3 cups of chopped roasted chicken
- 2 cups of shredded cheddar cheese
- 2 cups white of shredded cheddar cheese
- 3 cups of shredded parmesan cheese

Directions:

1. Oven: 350F
2. Be sure to rub butter or to spray with non-stick cooking spray.
3. In a bowl, put in all the cheese and mix well.
4. Microwave the cheese till it melts
5. Put in the chicken and toss thoroughly.
6. Put two tablespoons of the cheese chicken combo in a pile on the baking sheet. Be sure to leave space between piles.
7. Bake for 4-6 minutes. The moment they turn golden brown at the edges, take them off.
8. Serve hot.

Nutrition:
Calories: 387 kcal   **Fat:** 19.5 g   **Fiber:** 4.1 g   **Carbohydrates:** 3.9 g   **Protein:** 14.5 g

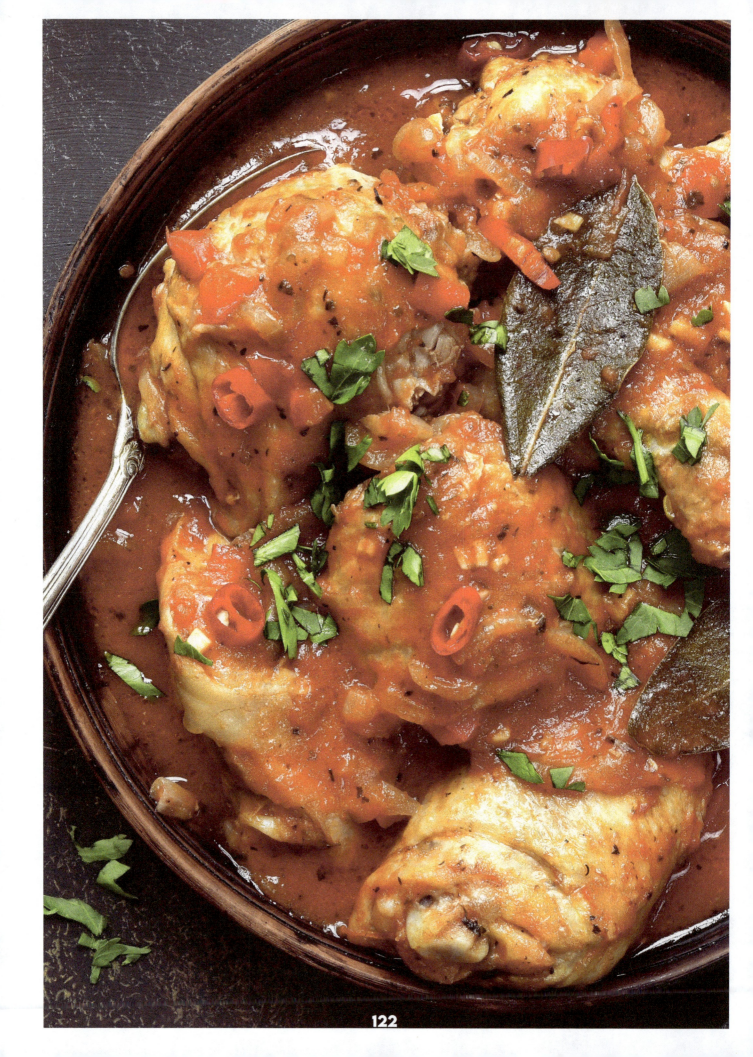

BRAISED CHICKEN IN ITALIAN TOMATO SAUCE

Prep Time: 15 min   **Cooking time:** 4 hrs.   **Servings:** 4

Ingredients:

- 1/4 cup olive oil, divided
- 4 (4-ounce / 113-g) boneless chicken thighs
- Pepper and salt
- 1/2 cup chicken stock
- 4 ounces (113 g) julienned oil-packed sun-dried tomatoes
- 1 (28-ounce / 794-g) can sodium-free diced tomatoes
- 2 tablespoons dried oregano
- 2 tablespoons minced garlic
- Red pepper flakes, to taste
- 2 tablespoons chopped fresh parsley

Directions:

1. Heat oil then put the chicken thighs in the skillet and sprinkle salt and black pepper to season.
2. Sear the chicken thighs for 10 minutes or until well browned.
3. Flip them halfway through the cooking time.
4. Put the chicken thighs, stock, tomatoes, oregano, garlic, and red pepper flakes into the slow cooker. Stir to coat the chicken thighs well.
5. High cook for 4 hrs.
6. Transfer the chicken thighs to four plates.
7. Pour the sauce which remains in the slow cooker over the chicken thighs and top with fresh parsley before serving warm.

Nutrition:
Calories: 464 kcal   **Fat:** 12.1 g   **Fiber:** 8.5 g   **Carbohydrates:** 6.4 g   **Protein:** 13.1 g

CHICKEN SPINACH SALAD

Prep Time: 15 min   **Cooking time:** 0 min   **Servings:** 3

Ingredients:

- 2 1/2 cups of spinach
- 4 1/2 ounces of boiled chicken
- 2 boiled eggs
- 1/2 cup of chopped cucumber
- 3 slices of bacon
- 1 small avocado
- 1 tablespoon olive oil
- 1/2 teaspoon of coconut oil
- Pinch of Salt
- Pepper

Directions:

1. Dice the boiled eggs.
2. Slice boiled chicken, bacon, avocado, spinach, cucumber, and combine them in a bowl. Then add diced boiled eggs.
3. Drizzle with some oil. Mix well.
4. Add salt and pepper to taste.
5. Enjoy.

Nutrition:
Calories: 265 kcal   **Fat:** 9.5 g   **Fiber:** 10.5 g   **Carbohydrates:** 3.3 g   **Protein:** 14.1 g

TURKEY BREAST WITH TOMATO-OLIVE SALSA

Prep Time: 20 min   **Cooking time:** 10 min   **Servings:** 4

Ingredients:

For turkey:
- 4 boneless turkey. Skinned.
- 3 tablespoons olive oil
- Salt
- Pepper

For salsa:
- 6 chopped tomatoes
- 1/2 diced onions
- 5 ounces of pitted and chopped olives
- 2 crushed garlic cloves
- 2 tablespoons of chopped basil
- 1 large diced jalapeno
- Pepper
- Salt

Directions:

1. In a bowl, put salt, pepper, and three spoons of oil, mix and coat the turkey with this mixture.
2. Place it on a preheated grill and grill for ten minutes.
3. In another bowl, mix garlic, olives, tomatoes, pepper, and drop the rest of the oil. Sprinkle salt and toss. Serve this salsa with turkey is warm.

Nutrition:
Calories: 387 kcal   **Fat:** 12.5 g   **Fiber:** 8.4 g   **Carbohydrates:** 3.1 g   **Protein:** 18.6 g

TURKEY MEATBALLS

Prep Time: 15 min   **Cooking time:** 20 min   **Servings:** 2

Ingredients:

- 1 pound of ground turkey
- 1 tablespoon of fish sauce
- 1 diced onion
- 2 tablespoons of soy sauce
- 1/2 almond flour
- 1/8 cup of ground beef
- 1/2 teaspoon of garlic powder
- 1/2 teaspoon of salt
- 1/2 teaspoon of ground ginger
- 1/2 teaspoon of thyme
- 1/2 teaspoon of curry
- 5 tablespoons of olive oil

Directions:

1. Combine ground turkey, fish sauce, one diced onion, soy sauce, ground beef, seasonings, oil, and flour in a large mixing bowl. Mix it thoroughly.
2. Form meatballs depending on preferred size.
3. Heat skillet and pour in 3 tablespoons of oil [you may need more depending on the size of meat balls].
4. Cook meatballs until evenly browned on each side. Serve hot.

Nutrition:
Calories: 281 kcal   **Fat:** 11.6 g   **Fiber:** 6.9 g   **Carbohydrates:** 4.6 g   **Protein:** 15.1 g

CHEESY BACON RANCH CHICKEN

Prep Time: 40 min **Cooking time:** 35 min **Servings:** 8

Ingredients:

- 8 boneless and skinned chicken breasts
- 1 cup of olive oil
- 8 thick slices bacon
- 3 cups of shredded mozzarella
- 1 1/4 tablespoon of ranch seasoning
- 1 small chopped onion
- Chopped chives
- Kosher salt or pink salt
- Black pepper

Directions:

1. Preheat skillet and heat little oil, and cook bacon evenly on both sides.
2. Save four tablespoons of drippings and put the others away.
3. Add in salt and pepper in a bowl and rub it over chicken to season.
4. Put 1/2 oil on the flame to cook the chicken from each side for 5 to 7 minutes.
5. When ready, reduce the heat and put in the ranch seasoning, then add mozzarella.
6. Cover and cook on a low flame for 3-5 minutes.
7. Put in bacon fat and chopped chives, then bacon and cover it.
8. Take off and serve warm.

Nutrition:
Calories: 387 kcal **Fat:** 15.1 g **Fiber:** 10.6 g **Carbohydrates:** 5.9 g **Protein:** 12.9 g

INDIAN BUTTERED CHICKEN

 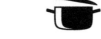

Prep Time: 15 min   **Cooking time:** 30 min   **Servings:** 4

Ingredients:

- 3 tablespoons unsalted butter
- 1 medium yellow onion, chopped
- 2 garlic cloves, minced
- 1 teaspoon fresh ginger, minced
- 1 1/2 pounds grass-fed chicken breasts, cut into 3/4-inch chunks
- 2 tomatoes, chopped finely
- 1 tablespoon garam masala
- 1 teaspoon red chili powder
- 1 teaspoon ground cumin
- Salt and ground black pepper, as required
- 1 cup heavy cream
- 2 tablespoons fresh cilantro, chopped

Directions:

1. In a wok, melt butter and sauté the onions for about 5–6 minutes.
2. Now, add in ginger and garlic and sauté for about 1 minute.
3. Add the tomatoes and cook for about 2–3 minutes, crushing with the back of the spoon.
4. Stir in the chicken spices, salt, and black pepper, and cook for about 6–8 minutes or until the desired doneness of the chicken.
5. Put in the cream and cook for about 8–10 more minutes, stirring occasionally.
6. Garnish with fresh cilantro and serve hot.

Nutrition:
Calories: 456 kcal   **Fat:** 14.1 g   **Fiber:** 10.5 g   **Carbohydrates:** 6.8 g   **Protein:** 12.8 g

BROCCOLI AND CHICKEN CASSEROLE

Prep Time: 15 min   **Cooking time:** 35 min   **Servings:** 6

Ingredients:

- 2 tablespoons butter
- 1/4 cup cooked bacon, crumbled
- 2 1/2 cups cheddar cheese, shredded and divided
- 4 ounces cream cheese, softened
- 1/4 cup heavy whipping cream
- 1/2 pack ranch seasoning mix
- 2/3 cup homemade chicken broth
- 1 1/2 cups small broccoli florets
- 2 cups cooked grass-fed chicken breast, shredded

Directions:

1. Preheat your oven to 350°F.
2. Arrange a rack in the upper portion of the oven.
3. For the chicken mixture: In a large wok, melt the butter over low heat.
4. Add the bacon, 1/2 cup of cheddar cheese, cream cheese, heavy whipping cream, ranch seasoning, and broth, and with a wire whisk, beat until well combined.
5. Cook for about 5 minutes, stirring frequently.
6. Meanwhile, in a microwave-safe dish, place the broccoli and microwave until desired tenderness is achieved.
7. In the wok, add the chicken and broccoli and mix until well combined.
8. Remove from the heat and transfer the mixture into a casserole dish.
9. Top the chicken mixture with the remaining cheddar cheese.
10. Bake for about 25 minutes.
11. Now, set the oven to broiler.
12. Broil the chicken mixture for about 2–3 minutes or until cheese is bubbly.
13. Serve hot.

Nutrition:
Calories: 431 kcal   **Fat:** 10.5 g   **Fiber:** 9.1 g   **Carbohydrates:** 4.9 g   **Protein:** 14.1 g

CHICKEN CAULIFLOWER FRIED RICE

Prep Time: 15 min   **Cooking time:** 20 min   **Servings:** 4

Ingredients:

- 1/2 teaspoon of sesame oil
- 1 small carrot (chopped)
- 1 tablespoon of avocado or coconut oil
- 1 small onion (finely sliced)
- 1/2 cup of snap peas (chopped)
- 1/2 cup of red peppers cut finely
- 1 tablespoon of garlic
- 1 tablespoon of garlic, properly chopped
- 1 teaspoon of salt
- 2 teaspoons of garlic powder
- 4 chicken breasts, chopped and cooked
- 4 cups of rice cauliflower
- 2 large scrambled eggs
- Gluten-free soy sauce, one quarter cup size

Directions:

1. Gently season the chicken breasts with 1/2 tablespoon of salt, 1/4 tablespoon of pepper, and 1/2 tablespoon of olive oil. Cook the chicken on any pan of your choice
2. Add coconut/olive/avocado oil. Cut some onions and carrots and sauce and leave for up to 3 minutes
3. Next, add the rest of the vegetables, pepper/salt/garlic powder and then cook for extra 3 minutes
4. Put in fresh garlic coconut aminos or soy sauce and riced cauliflower; then stir
5. Add scrambled eggs and chicken and mix until they are well combined
6. Put off the heat and then stir in some green peas. Season again. You can top it with sesame seeds if you like

Nutrition:
Calories: 271 kcal   **Fat:** 15.1 g   **Fiber:** 12.4 g   **Carbohydrates:** 3.9 g   **Protein:** 5.1 g

CHICKEN PARMIGIANA

Prep Time: 15 min　　**Cooking time:** 25 min　　**Servings:** 5

Ingredients:

- 5 (6-ounce) grass-fed skinless, boneless chicken breasts
- 1 large organic egg, beaten
- 1/2 cup superfine blanched almond flour
- 1/4 cup Parmesan cheese, grated
- 1/2 teaspoon dried parsley
- 1/2 teaspoon paprika
- 1/2 teaspoon garlic powder
- Salt and ground black pepper, as required
- 1/4 cup olive oil
- 1 cup sugar-free tomato sauce
- 5 ounces mozzarella cheese, thinly sliced
- 2 tablespoons fresh parsley, chopped

Directions:

1. Preheat your oven to 375°F.
2. Arrange one chicken breast between 2 pieces of parchment paper.
3. With a meat mallet, pound the chicken breast into a 1/2-inch thickness
4. Repeat with the remaining chicken breasts.
5. Add the beaten egg into a shallow dish.
6. Place the almond flour, Parmesan, parsley, spices, salt, and black pepper in another shallow dish, and mix well.
7. Dip chicken breasts into the whipped egg and then coat with the flour mixture.
8. Heat the oil in a deep wok over medium-high heat and fry the chicken breasts for about 3 minutes per side.
9. The chicken breasts must be transferred onto a paper towel-lined plate to drain.
10. At the bottom of a casserole, place about 1/2 cup of tomato sauce and spread evenly.
11. Arrange the chicken breasts over marinara sauce in a single layer.
12. Put sauce on top plus the mozzarella cheese slices.
13. Bake for about 20 minutes or until done completely.
14. Remove from the oven and serve hot with the garnishing of parsley.

Nutrition:
Calories: 398 kcal　**Fat:** 15.1 g　**Fiber:** 9.4 g　**Carbohydrates:** 4.1 g　**Protein:** 15.1 g

GREEK STUFFED CHICKEN BREAST

Prep Time: 30 min   **Cooking time:** 30 min   **Servings:** 4

Ingredients:

- 1 tablespoon butter
- 1/4 cup chopped sweet onion
- 1/2 cup goat cheese, at room temperature
- 1/4 cup Kalamata olives, chopped
- 1/4 cup chopped roasted red pepper
- 2 tablespoons chopped fresh basil
- 4 (5-ounce) chicken breasts, skin-on
- 2 tablespoons extra-virgin olive oil

Directions:

1. Preheat the oven to 400°F.
2. Melt some butter and add the onion. Sauté until tender, about 3 minutes.
3. The onion must be added to a bowl then continue putting cheese, olives, red pepper, and basil. Stir until well blended, then refrigerate for about 30 minutes.
4. Cut horizontal pockets into each chicken breast, and stuff them evenly with the filling. Secure the two sides of each breast with toothpicks.
5. Heat oil in a preheated pan. The chicken must be browned per side.
6. Roast in the oven for 15 minutes. Remove the toothpicks and serve.

Nutrition:
Calories: 381 kcal   **Fat:** 15.9 g   **Fiber:** 5.4 g   **Carbohydrates:** 3.9 g   **Protein:** 14.1 g

CHICKEN MEATLOAF CUPS WITH PANCETTA

Prep Time: 15 min   **Cooking time:** 30 min   **Servings:** 6

Ingredients:

- 2 tbsp. onion, chopped
- 1 tsp. garlic, minced
- 1-pound ground chicken
- 2 ounces cooked pancetta, chopped
- 1 egg, beaten
- 1 tsp. mustard
- Salt and black pepper, to taste
- 1/2 tsp. crushed red pepper flakes
- 1 tsp. dried basil
- 1/2 tsp. dried oregano
- 4 ounces cheddar cheese, cubed

Directions:

1. In a mixing bowl, mix mustard, onion, ground turkey, egg, bacon, and garlic. Season with oregano, red pepper, black pepper, basil, and salt.
2. Split the mixture into muffin cups—lower one cube of cheddar cheese into each meatloaf cup.
3. Close the top to cover the cheese.
4. Bake in the oven at 345°F for 20 minutes, or until the meatloaf cups become golden brown.

Nutrition:
Calories: 231 kcal   **Fat:** 10.4 g   **Fiber:** 5.1 g   **Carbohydrates:** 3.9 g   **Protein:** 11.4 g

CHICKEN SCHNITZEL

 Prep Time: 15 min   **Cooking time:** 20 min   **Servings:** 4

Ingredients:

- 1 tbsp. chopped fresh parsley
- 4 garlic cloves, minced
- 1 tbsp. plain vinegar
- 1 tbsp. coconut aminos
- 2 tsp. sugar-free maple syrup
- 2 tsp. chili pepper
- Salt and black pepper to taste
- 6 tbsp. coconut oil
- 1 lb. asparagus, stiff stems removed
- 4 chicken breasts, skin-on and boneless
- 2 cups grated Mexican cheese blend
- 1 tbsp. mixed sesame seeds
- 1 cup almond flour
- 4 eggs, beaten
- 6 tbsp. avocado oil
- 1 tsp. chili flakes for garnish

Directions:

1. In a bowl, whisk the parsley, garlic, vinegar, coconut aminos, maple syrup, chili pepper, salt, and black pepper. Set aside.
2. Heat the coconut oil in a large skillet and stir-fry the asparagus for 8 to 10 minutes or until tender. Remove the asparagus into a large bowl and toss with the vinegar mixture. Set aside for serving.
3. Cover the chicken breasts in plastic wraps and use a meat tenderizer to pound the chicken until flattened to 2-inch thickness gently.
4. On a plate, mix the Mexican cheese blend and sesame seeds. Dredge the chicken pieces in the almond flour, dip in the egg on both sides, and generously coat in the seed mix.
5. Heat the avocado oil. Cook the chicken until golden brown and cooked within.
6. Divide the asparagus onto four serving plates, place a chicken on each, and garnish with the chili flakes. Serve warm.

Nutrition:
Calories: 451 kcal   **Fat:** 18.5 g   **Fiber:** 12.9 g   **Carbohydrates:** 5.9 g   **Protein:** 19.5 g

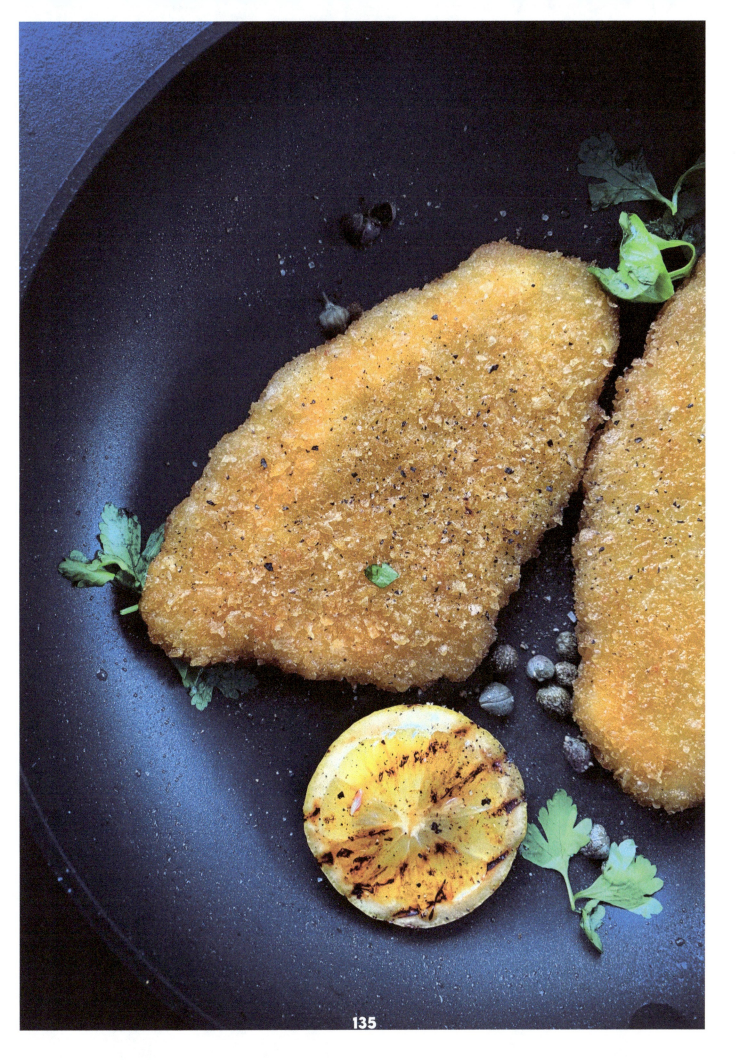

THAI PEANUT CHICKEN SKEWERS

Prep Time: 10 min **Cooking time:** 15 min **Servings:** 2

Ingredients:

- 1-pound boneless skinless chicken breast, cut into chunks
- 3 tablespoons coconut aminos
- 1/2 teaspoon Sriracha sauce, plus 1/4 teaspoon
- 3 teaspoons toasted sesame oil, divided
- Ghee, for oiling
- 2 tablespoons peanut butter
- Pink Himalayan salt
- Freshly ground black pepper

Directions:

1. In a bag, combine the chicken chunks with two tablespoons of soy sauce, 1/2 teaspoon of Sriracha sauce, and two teaspoons of sesame oil. Marinate the chicken.
2. If you are using wood 8-inch skewers, soak them in water for 30 minutes before using.
3. Oil the grill pan with ghee.
4. Thread the chicken chunks onto the skewers.
5. Cook the skewers over low heat for 10 to 15 minutes, flipping halfway through.
6. Meanwhile, mix the peanut dipping sauce.
7. Stir together the remaining one tablespoon of soy sauce, 1/4 teaspoon of Sriracha sauce, one teaspoon of sesame oil, and the peanut butter.
8. Season with pink Himalayan salt and pepper.
9. Serve the chicken skewers with a small dish of the peanut sauce.

Nutrition:
Calories: 390 kcal **Fat:** 18.4 g **Fiber:** 12.9 g **Carbohydrates:** 2.1 g **Protein:** 17.4 g

CHICKEN POT PIE

 Prep Time: 15 min   **Cooking time:** 25 min   **Servings:** 4

Ingredients:

- For the filling
- 1/2 medium onion, chopped
- 2 celery stalks, chopped
- 1/2 cup fresh or frozen peas
- 2 tablespoons butter
- 1 garlic clove, minced
- 11/2 pounds chicken thighs
- 1 cup chicken broth
- 1/2 cup heavy (whipping) cream
- 1/2 cup shredded low-moisture mozzarella cheese
- 1 teaspoon dried thyme
- 1/2 teaspoon pink Himalayan sea salt
- 1/2 teaspoon freshly ground black pepper
- For the crust
- 1 cup almond flour
- 2 tablespoons butter, at room temperature
- 2 tablespoons sour cream
- 1 large egg white
- 1 tablespoon ground flaxseed
- 1 teaspoon xanthan gum
- 1 teaspoon baking powder
- 1/2 teaspoon garlic powder
- 1/4 teaspoon pink Himalayan sea salt
- 1/4 teaspoon dried thyme

Directions:

1. Filling: In a saucepan, combine the onion, celery, peas, butter, and garlic over medium heat.
2. Cook for about 5 minutes, until the onion starts to turn translucent.
3. In a large skillet, cook the chicken thighs for 3 to 5 minutes, until there is no more visible pink. Add the cooked chicken and all juices to the pan with the vegetables.
4. Add the broth, cream, mozzarella, thyme, salt, and pepper to the pan. Simmer it until sauce thickens, stirring occasionally.
5. Preheat the oven to 400°F.
6. In a bowl or container, combine the almond flour, butter, sour cream, egg white, flaxseed, xanthan gum, baking powder, garlic powder, salt, and thyme.
7. Form this into a dough.
8. Place the dough between 2 sheets of parchment paper and roll out into a 10-inch round that is 1/4 inch thick.
9. Fill an 8-inch pie pan or 4 (6-ounce) ramekins with the chicken filling.
10. Top the pie pan with the crust, flipping it onto the filling and peeling away the parchment paper. If using ramekins, cut circles of the dough and fit them onto the ramekins.
11. Pinch to seal the edges, and trim off any excess.
12. Baking time: 10-12 minutes
13. Let cool for 5 minutes, then serve.

Nutrition:
Calories: 341 kcal   **Fat:** 18.4 g   **Fiber:** 10.3 g   **Carbohydrates:** 4.1 g   **Protein:** 12.5 g

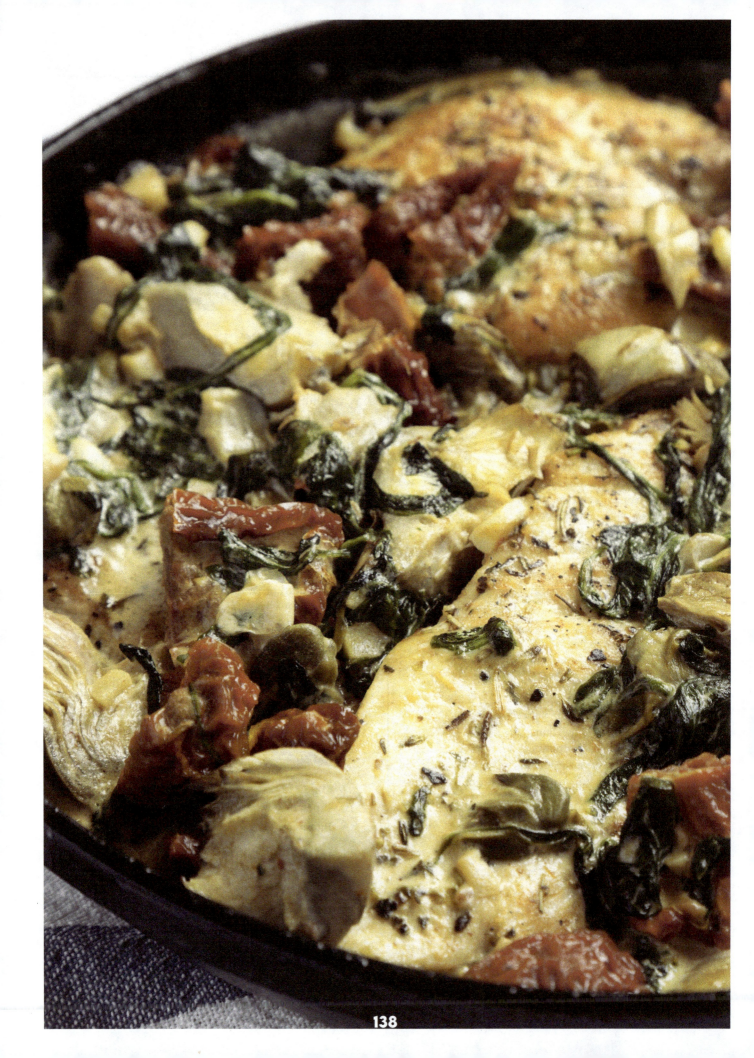

TUSCAN CHICKEN

 Prep Time: 15 min

 Cooking time: 15 min

 Servings: 6

Ingredients:

- 1 1/2 pounds chicken breasts, pasteurized, skinless, thinly sliced
- 1/2 cup sun-dried tomatoes
- 1 cup spinach, chopped
- 1 teaspoon garlic powder
- 1 teaspoon Italian seasoning
- 2 tablespoons avocado oil
- 1/2 cup grated parmesan cheese
- 1 cup heavy cream, full-fat
- 1/2 cup chicken broth, pasteurized

Directions:

1. Take a large skillet pan, place it over medium-high heat, add oil, and when hot, add chicken and then cook for 3–5 minutes per side until golden brown.
2. Add garlic powder, Italian seasoning, and cheese into the pan, pour in the broth and cream, and then whisk until combined.
3. Switch heat to medium-high, cook the sauce for 2 minutes until it begins to thicken, then add tomatoes and spinach and simmer until spinach leaves begin to wilt.
4. Return chicken to the pan, toss until mixed, and cook for 2 minutes until hot.
5. Serve chicken with cooked Keto pasta, such as zucchini noodles.

Nutrition:
Calories: 390 kcal **Fat:** 16.1 g **Fiber:** 12.8 g **Carbohydrates:** 3 g **Protein:** 19 g

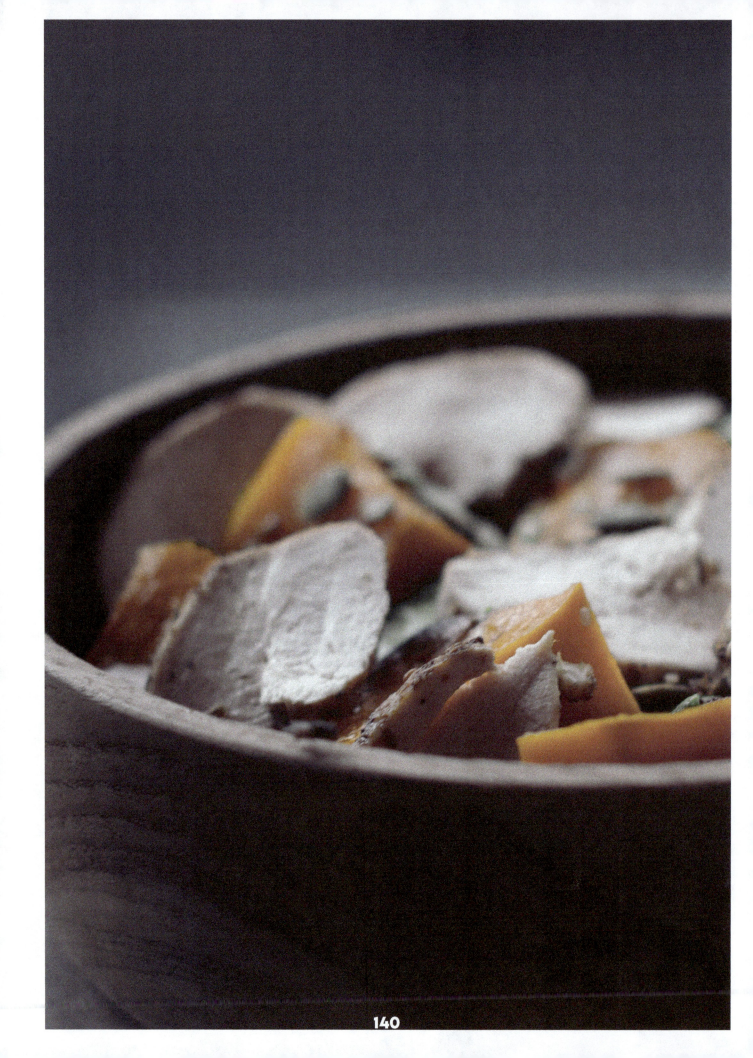

THAI CHICKEN SALAD BOWL

 Prep Time: 12 min   **Cooking time:** 15 min   **Servings:** 2

Ingredients:

Marinade:
- 1 clove garlic, minced
- 1 tbsp. grated ginger
- 1 small red chili, finely chopped
- 1/2 stalk lemongrass, finely chopped
- 2 tbsp. fresh lime juice
- 1 tsp. fish sauce
- 1 tbsp. coconut aminos
- Salad:
- 8 oz (226g) (2-pieces) chicken breasts
- 1/2 cup shredded red cabbage
- 1/2 cup shredded green cabbage
- 2/3 cup grated carrot
- 1 tbsp. chopped mint
- 1/2 cup chopped cilantro
- 1 tbsp. chopped chives
- 1/4 cup blanched almonds

Dressing:
- 3 tbsp. extra virgin olive oil
- Salt and pepper, to taste

Directions:

1. Oven: 400 F
2. Combine the garlic, ginger, red chili, lemongrass, lime juice, fish sauce, and coconut aminos in a bowl for marinating and crush with a mortar.
3. Flatten the chicken breasts with a meat mallet.
4. Add the chicken in a bowl and add half of the marinade, and coat the chicken evenly.
5. Make it cool in the refrigerator for a maximum of 30 minutes or an hour.
6. Combine both cabbages, carrot, mint, cilantro, and chives in a bowl.
7. In a baking tray, spread out the almonds and roast in the oven for 5-8 minutes, set aside.
8. Grill the chicken in a griddle.
9. Cook through then slice.
10. Mix int the remaining ingredients.

Nutrition:
Calories: 351 kcal **Fat:** 15.7 g **Fiber:** 11.4 g **Carbohydrates:** 3.1 g **Protein:** 12.5 g

CHICKEN QUESADILLA

Prep Time: 15 min   **Cooking time:** 25 min   **Servings:** 4

Ingredients:

- 1 tbsp. extra-virgin olive oil
- 1 bell pepper, sliced
- 1/2 yellow onion, sliced
- 1/2 tsp. chili powder
- Kosher salt
- Freshly ground black pepper
- 3 c. shredded Monterey Jack
- 3 c. shredded cheddar
- 4 c. shredded chicken
- 1 avocado, thinly sliced
- 1 green onion, thinly sliced
- Sour cream, for serving

Directions:

1. Let the oven preheat to 400F.
2. Prepare two baking sheets with a baking mat or parchment paper.
3. Heat oil.
4. Put pepper and onion and season with chili powder, salt, and pepper.
5. Cook until soft, 5 minutes. Transfer to a plate.
6. In a medium bowl, stir together cheeses.
7. Put 1 1/2 cups of cheese mixture onto both prepared baking sheets centers.
8. Spread the cheese evenly in a circle shape, like a flour tortilla.
9. Bake the quesadilla for about 20 minutes.
10. Put onion-pepper mixture, shredded chicken, and avocado slices to one half of each.
11. Let cool slightly.
12. Then use the parchment paper and a little spatula to gently lift.
13. Fold the cheese tortillas empty side over the filling side.
14. Place the quesadilla baking sheet in the oven to heat, 3 to 5 minutes more.
15. Decorate with green onion and sour cream and serve.

Nutrition:
Calories: 299 kcal   **Fat:** 12.1 g   **Fiber:** 4.1 g   **Carbohydrates:** 4.1 g   **Protein:** 10.1 g

CHICKEN ROLLATINI

Prep Time: 15 min   **Cooking time:** 30 min   **Servings:** 4

Ingredients:

- 4 (3-ounce) boneless skinless chicken breasts, pounded to about 1/3 inch thick
- 4 ounces ricotta cheese
- 4 slices prosciutto (4 ounces)
- 1 cup fresh spinach
- 1/2 cup almond flour
- 1/2 cup grated Parmesan cheese
- 2 eggs, beaten
- 1/4 cup good-quality olive oil

Directions:

1. Preheat the oven. Set the oven temperature to 400°F.
2. Prepare the chicken—Pat the chicken breasts dry with paper towels. Spread 1/4 of the ricotta in the middle of each breast.
3. Place the prosciutto over the ricotta and 1/4 cup of the spinach on the prosciutto.
4. Fold the long edges of the chicken breast over the filling, then roll the chicken breast up to enclose the filling.
5. Place the rolls seam-side down on your work surface.
6. Bread the chicken. On a plate, stir together the almond flour and Parmesan and set it next to the beaten eggs.
7. Carefully dip a chicken roll in the egg, then roll it in the almond-flour mixture until it is completely covered.
8. Set the rolls seam-side down on your work surface. Repeat with the other rolls.
9. Brown the rolls. In a medium skillet over medium heat, warm the olive oil.
10. Place the rolls seam-side down in the skillet and brown them on all sides, turning them carefully, about 10 minutes in total.
11. Transfer the rolls, seam-side down, to a 9-by-9-inch baking dish—Bake the chicken rolls for 25 minutes, or until they're cooked through.
12. Serve. Place one chicken roll on each of four plates and serve them immediately.

Nutrition:
Calories: 365 kcal   **Fat:** 17.1 g   **Fiber:** 9.4 g   **Carbohydrates:** 3.2 g   **Protein:** 1.4 g

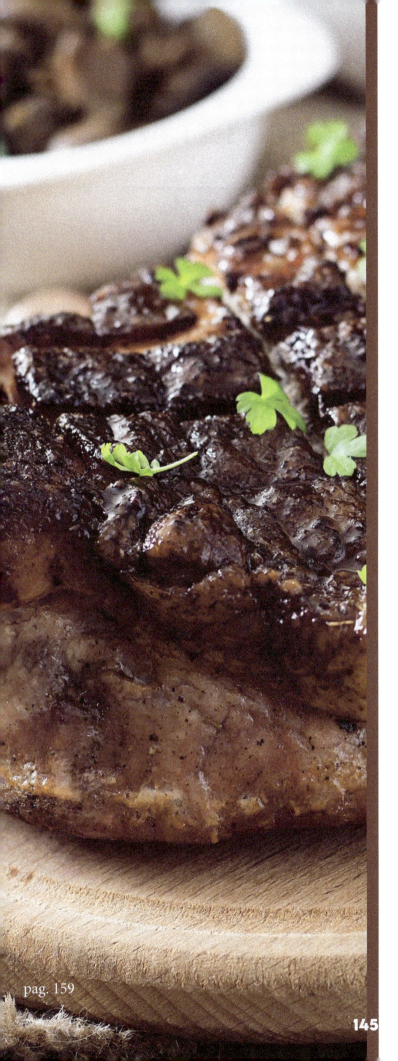

14

MEAT RECIPES

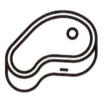

BEEF SHANKS BRAISED IN RED WINE SAUCE

Prep Time: 20 min   **Cooking time:** 8 hrs   **Servings:** 6

Ingredients:

- 2 tablespoons olive oil
- 2 pounds (907 g) beef shanks
- 2 cups dry red wine
- 3 cups beef stock
- 1 sprig of fresh rosemary
- 5 garlic cloves, finely chopped
- 1 onion, finely chopped
- Pepper and salt

Directions:

1. Heat olive oil.
2. Put the beef shanks into the skillet and fry for 5 to 10 minutes until well browned.
3. the beef shanks halfway through. Set aside.
4. The red wine must be poured into the pot and let it simmer.
5. Add the cooked beef shanks, dry red wine, beef stock, rosemary, garlic, onion, salt, and black pepper to the slow cooker. Stir to mix well.
6. Slow cook with the lid on for 8 hrs.

Nutrition:
Calories: 341 kcal   **Fat:** 19.6 g   **Fiber:** 10 g   **Carbohydrates:** 15.4 g   **Protein:** 21.6 g

HERBED GRILLED LAMB

Prep Time: 15 min **Cooking time:** 20 min **Servings:** 6

Ingredients:

- 2 pounds of lamb
- 5 spoons of ghee butter
- 3 tablespoons of Keto mustard
- 2 minced garlic cloves
- 1 1/2 tablespoon of chopped basil
- 1/2 tablespoon of pepper
- 3 tablespoons of olive oil
- 1/2 teaspoon of salt

Directions:

1. Mix butter, mustard, and basil with a pinch of salt to taste. Then, set aside.
2. Mix garlic, salt, and pepper together. Then, add a teaspoon of oil.
3. Season the lamb generously with this mix.
4. Grill the lamb on medium heat until fully cooked.
5. Take butter mix and spread generously on chops and serve hot.

Nutrition:
Calories: 390 kcal **Fat:** 19.5 g **Fiber:** 5.9 g **Carbohydrates:** 3.2 g **Protein:** 18.6 g

CHEESY BACON SQUASH SPAGHETTI

 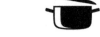

Prep Time: 30 min   **Cooking time:** 50 min   **Servings:** 4

Ingredients:

- 2 pounds spaghetti squash
- 2 pounds bacon
- 1/2 cup of butter
- 2 cups of shredded parmesan cheese
- Salt
- Black pepper

Directions:

1. Let the oven preheat to 375F.
2. Trim or remove each stem of spaghetti squash, slice into rings no more than an inch wide, and take out the seeds.
3. Lay the sliced rings down on the baking sheet, bake for 40-45 minutes.
4. It is ready when the strands separate easily when a fork is used to scrape it. Let it cool.
5. Cook sliced up bacon until crispy. Take out and let it cool.
6. Take off the shell on each ring, separate each strand with a fork, and put them in a bowl.
7. Heat the strands in a microwave to get them warm, then put in butter and stir around till the butter melts.
8. Pour in parmesan cheese and bacon crumbles, and add salt and pepper to your taste.
9. Enjoy.

Nutrition:
Calories: 398 kcal   **Fat:** 12.5 g   **Fiber:** 9.4 g   **Carbohydrates:** 4.1 g   **Protein:** 5.1 g

STUFFED ONIONS

Prep Time: 35 min   **Cooking time:** 45 min   **Servings:** 5

Ingredients:

- 5 onions (medium-sized)
- 3/4 pound of ground beef
- 2 medium eggs
- Italian seasoning to taste
- 2 spoons of olive oil
- Salt
- Black pepper
- 1/4 cup of ground pork
- 4 tablespoons parmesan cheese
- Worcestershire sauce to taste
- 2 ounces of quartered cheddar cheese

Directions:

1. Preheat oven to 350°F.
2. Take out the inner layers, so the onion is hollow and bottomless. Place it in a casserole dish.
3. In another bowl, whisk eggs lightly.
4. In another bowl, mix the two kinds of cheese.
5. In another bowl, put in the ground beef, egg mixture, olive oil, ground pork, and Worcestershire sauce, 1/4 teaspoon of salt and other seasonings to taste, and mix well.
6. Fully stuff each onion with the mix of beef and egg.
7. Make a space in the stuffing for cheese balls and put inside.
8. Cover the onion with another meat layer, and bake for 30-45 minutes.

Nutrition:
Calories: 299 kcal   **Fat:** 12.6 g   **Fiber:** 5.9 g   **Carbohydrates:** 4.9 g   **Protein:** 16.7 g

SHEPHERD'S PIE

Prep Time: 5 min   **Cooking time:** 3/9 min   **Servings:** 2

Ingredients:

- 1/4 cup olive oil
- 1-pound grass-fed ground beef
- 1/2 cup celery, chopped
- 1/4 cup yellow onion, chopped
- 3 garlic cloves, minced
- 1 cup tomatoes, chopped
- 2 (12-ounce) packages riced cauliflower, cooked and well-drained
- 1 cup cheddar cheese, shredded
- 1/4 cup Parmesan cheese, shredded
- 1 cup heavy cream
- 1 teaspoon dried thyme

Directions:

1. Preheat your oven to 350°F.
2. Heat oil heat and cook the ground beef, celery, onions, and garlic for about 8–10 minutes.
3. Immediately stir in the tomatoes.
4. Transfer mixture into a 10x7-inch casserole dish evenly.
5. In a food processor, add the cauliflower, cheeses, cream, thyme, and pulse until a mashed potatoes-like mixture is formed.
6. Spread the cauliflower mixture over the meat in the casserole dish evenly.
7. Bake for about 35–40 minutes.
8. Cut into desired sized pieces and serve.

Nutrition:
Calories: 387 kcal   **Fat:** 11.5 g   **Fiber:** 9.4 g   **Carbohydrates:** 5.5 g   **Protein:** 18.5 g

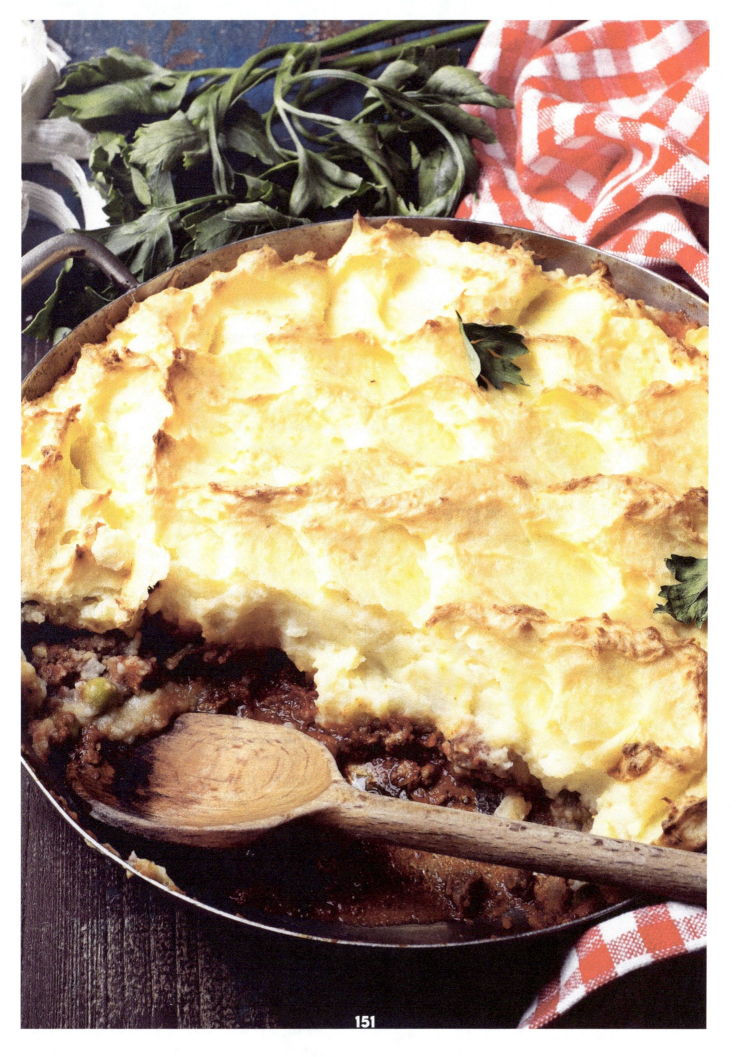

BEEF WELLINGTON

Prep Time: 20 min   **Cooking time:** 40 min   **Servings:** 4

Ingredients:

- 2 (4-ounce) grass-fed beef tenderloin steaks, halved
- Salt and ground black pepper, as required
- 1 tablespoon butter
- 1 cup mozzarella cheese, shredded
- 1/2 cup almond flour
- 4 tablespoons liver pate

Directions:

1. Preheat your oven to 400°F.
2. Grease a baking sheet.
3. Season the steaks with pepper and salt.
4. Sear the beef steaks for about 2–3 minutes per side.
5. In a microwave-safe bowl, add the mozzarella cheese and microwave for about 1 minute.
6. Remove from the microwave and stir in the almond flour until a dough forms.
7. Place the dough between 2 parchment paper pieces and, with a rolling pin, roll to flatten it.
8. Remove the upper parchment paper piece.
9. Divide the rolled dough into four pieces.
10. Place one tablespoon of pate onto each dough piece and top with one steak piece.
11. Cover each steak piece with dough completely.
12. Arrange the covered steak pieces onto the prepared baking sheet in a single layer.
13. Baking time: 20-30 minutes
14. Serve warm.

Nutrition:
Calories: 412 kcal   **Fat:** 15.6 g   **Fiber:** 9.1 g   **Carbohydrates:** 4.9 g   **Protein:** 18.5 g

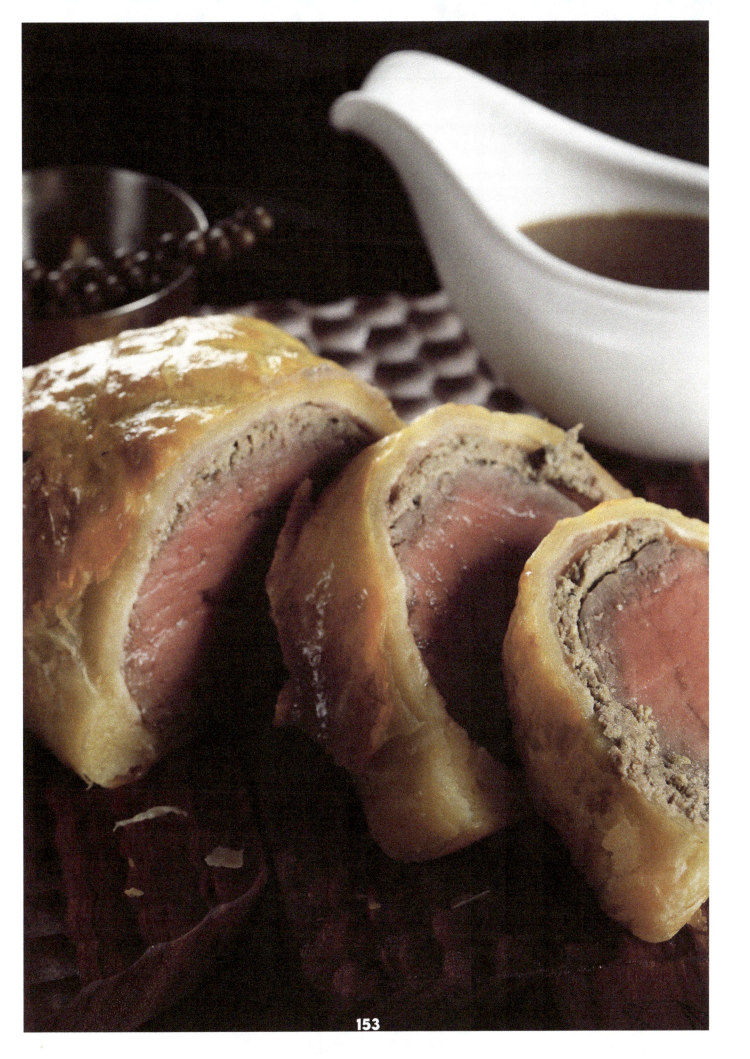

STICKY PORK RIBS

Prep Time: 25 min **Cooking time:** 90 min **Servings:** 8

Ingredients:

- 1/4 cups granulated erythritol
- 1 tablespoon garlic powder
- 1 tablespoon paprika
- 1/2 teaspoon red chili powder
- 4 pounds pork ribs, membrane removed
- Salt and ground black pepper, as required
- 1 1/2 teaspoons liquid smoke
- 1 1/2 cups sugar-free BBQ sauce

Directions:

1. Preheat your oven to 300°F.
2. In a bowl, mix well erythritol, garlic powder, paprika, and chili powder.
3. Season the ribs with pepper and salt. And then coat with the liquid smoke.
4. Now, rub the ribs evenly with erythritol mixture.
5. Arrange ribs onto the prepared baking sheet, meaty side down.
6. Arrange two layers of foil on top of ribs and then roll and crimp edges tightly.
7. Bake for about 2–2 1/2 hours or until the desired doneness.
8. Now, set the oven to broiler.
9. With a sharp knife, cut the ribs into serving-sized portions and evenly coat with the barbecue sauce.
10. Arrange the ribs onto a broiler pan, bony side up.
11. Broil for about 1–2 minutes per side.
12. Remove from the oven and serve hot.

Nutrition:
Calories: 415 kcal **Fat:** 18.1 g **Fiber:** 12.5 g **Carbohydrates:** 3.1 g **Protein:** 18.5 g

CREAMY PORK AND CELERIAC GRATIN

Prep Time: 20 min   **Cooking time:** 60 min   **Servings:** 4

Ingredients:

- 1/2 lb. celeriac, peeled and thinly sliced
- 1/3 cup almond milk
- 1/2 cup heavy cream
- 1/4 tsp. nutmeg powder
- Salt and black pepper to taste
- 1 tbsp. olive oil
- 1 lb. ground pork
- 1/2 medium white onion, chopped
- 1 garlic clove, minced
- 1/2 tsp. unsweetened tomato paste
- 3 tbsp. butter for greasing
- 1 cup crumbled queso fresco cheese
- 1 tbsp. chopped fresh parsley for garnish

Directions:

1. Let the oven preheat to 375F.
2. In a saucepan, add the celeriac, almond milk, heavy cream, nutmeg powder, and salt.
3. Cook until the celeriac softens. Drain afterward and set aside.
4. Heat oil and cook the pork for 5 minutes or starting to brown—season with salt and black pepper.
5. Stir in the onion, garlic, and cook for 5 minutes or until the onions soften.
6. The tomato paste must be added and continue cooking.
7. Grease a baking dish and lay half of the celeriac on the bottom of the dish.
8. Spread the tomato-pork sauce on top and cover with the remaining celeriac.
9. Finish the topping with the queso fresco cheese.
10. Let the gratin bake for about 45 minutes or until the cheese melts and is golden brown.
11. Remove from the oven to cool for 5 to 10 minutes, garnish with the parsley, and serve afterward.

Nutrition:
Calories: 486 kcal   **Fat:** 19.4 g   **Fiber:** 10.3 g   **Carbohydrates:** 8.5 g   **Protein:** 19.2 g

BBQ PULLED BEEF

 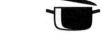

Prep Time: 15 min   **Cooking time:** 6 hrs   **Servings:** 10

Ingredients:

- 3 lbs. boneless chuck roast
- 2 tablespoons of salt
- 2 tablespoon of garlic powder
- 1 tablespoon of onion powder
- 1/4 apple cider vinegar
- 2 tablespoons of coconut aminos
- 1/2 cup of bone broth
- 1/4 cup of melted butter
- 1 tablespoon of black pepper
- 1 tablespoon of smoked paprika
- 2 tablespoon of tomato paste

Directions:

1. Mix salt, onion, paprika, black pepper, and garlic.
2. Next is to rub the mixture on the beef and then put the beef in a slow cooker
3. Use another bowl to melt butter. Then, add a tomato paste, coconut aminos, and vinegar.
4. Pour it all over the beef. Next is to add the bone broth into the slow cooker by pouring it around the beef
5. Cook for about 6 hrs.
6. After that, take out the beef and increase the temperature of the cooker so that the sauce can thicken. Tear the beef before adding it to the slow cooker and toss with the sauce.

Nutrition:
Calories: 315 kcal   **Fat:** 17 g   **Fiber:** 11.9 g   **Carbohydrates:** 4.1 g   **Protein:** 18.9 g

NUT-STUFFED PORK CHOPS

 Prep Time: 20 min   **Cooking time:** 30 min   **Servings:** 4

Ingredients:

- 3 ounces goat cheese
- 1/2 cup chopped walnuts
- 1/4 cup toasted chopped almonds
- 1 teaspoon chopped fresh thyme
- 4 center-cut pork chops, butterflied
- Sea salt
- Freshly ground black pepper
- 2 tablespoons olive oil

Directions:

1. Preheat the oven to 400°F.
2. In a container, stir together the goat cheese, walnuts, almonds, and thyme until well mixed.
3. Season the pork chops inside and outside with salt and pepper.
4. Stuff each chop, pushing the filling to the bottom of the cut section.
5. Secure the stuffing with toothpicks through the meat.
6. Heat oil. Pan sear the pork chops until they're browned on each side, about 10 minutes in total.
7. Put the pork chops into a baking dish and roast the chops in the oven until cooked through about 20 minutes.
8. Serve after removing the toothpicks.

Nutrition:
Calories: 425 kcal   **Fat:** 19.5 g   **Fiber:** 7.9 g   **Carbohydrates:** 6.5 g   **Protein:** 19.4 g

ROASTED PORK LOIN WITH BROWN MUSTARD SAUCE

Prep Time: 10 min **Cooking time:** 70 min **Servings:** 8

Ingredients:

- 1 (2-pound) boneless pork loin roast
- Sea salt
- Freshly ground black pepper
- 3 tablespoons olive oil
- 1 1/2 cups decadent (whipping) cream
- 3 tablespoons grainy mustard, such as Pommery

Directions:

1. Preheat the oven to 375°F.
2. Season the pork roast all over with sea salt and pepper.
3. Heat oil then all the sides of the roast must be browned, about 6 minutes in total, and place the roast in a baking dish.
4. When there are approximately 15 minutes of roasting time left, place a small saucepan over medium heat and add the heavy cream and mustard.
5. Stir the sauce until it simmers, then reduce the heat to low. Simmer the sauce until it is vibrant and thick, about 5 minutes. Remove the pan from the heat and set aside.

Nutrition:
Calories: 415 kcal   **Fat:** 18.4 g   **Fiber:** 11.3 g   **Carbohydrates:** 3.1 g   **Protein:** 17.4 g

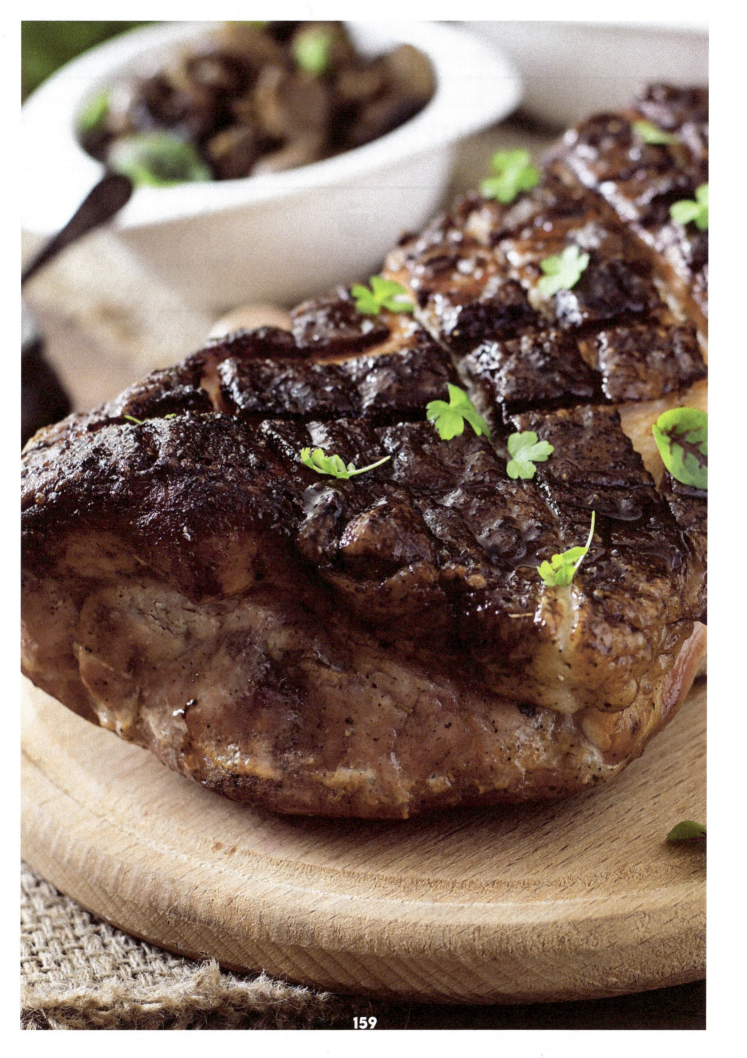

LAMB CHOPS WITH TAPENADE

Prep Time: 15 min **Cooking time:** 25 min **Servings:** 4

Ingredients:

FOR THE TAPENADE

- 1 cup pitted Kalamata olive
- 2 tablespoons chopped fresh parsley
- 2 tablespoons extra-virgin olive oil
- 2 teaspoons minced garlic
- 2 teaspoons freshly squeezed lemon juice

FOR THE LAMB CHOPS

- 2 (1-pound) racks French-cut lamb chops (8 bones each)
- Sea salt
- Freshly ground black pepper
- 1 tablespoon olive oil

Directions:

TO MAKE THE TAPENADE

1. Place the olives, parsley, olive oil, garlic, and lemon juice in a food processor and process until the mixture is puréed but still slightly chunky.
2. Transfer the tapenade to a container and store it sealed in the refrigerator until needed.

TO MAKE THE LAMB CHOPS

3. Preheat the oven to 450°F.
4. Season the lamb racks with pepper and salt
5. Heat oil
6. Pan sear the lamb racks on all sides until browned, about 5 minutes in total.
7. Arrange the racks upright in the skillet, with the bones interlaced, and roast them for about 20 minutes for medium-rare or until the internal temperature reaches 125°F.

Nutrition:
Calories: 387 kcal   **Fat:** 17.4 g   **Fiber:** 12.1 g   **Carbohydrates:** 5.4 g   **Protein:** 18.9 g

SESAME PORK WITH GREEN BEANS

Prep Time: 5 min   **Cooking time:** 10 min   **Servings:** 2

Ingredients:

- 2 boneless pork chops
- Pink Himalayan salt
- Freshly ground black pepper
- 2 tablespoons toasted sesame oil, divided
- 2 tablespoons soy sauce
- 1 teaspoon Sriracha sauce
- 1 cup fresh green beans

Directions:

1. On a cutting board, pat the pork chops dry with a paper towel. Slice the chops into strips and season with pink Himalayan salt and pepper.
2. In a large skillet over medium heat, heat one tablespoon of sesame oil.
3. Add the pork strips and cook them for 7 minutes, stirring occasionally.
4. In a small bowl, mix the remaining one tablespoon of sesame oil, the soy sauce, and the Sriracha sauce. Pour into the skillet with the pork.
5. Add the green beans to the skillet, reduce the heat to medium-low, and simmer for 3 to 5 minutes.
6. Divide the pork, green beans, and sauce between two wide, shallow bowls and serve.

Nutrition:
Calories: 387 kcal   **Fat:** 15.1 g   **Fiber:** 10 g   **Carbohydrates:** 4.1 g   **Protein:** 18.1 g

KALUA PORK WITH CABBAGE

 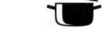

Prep Time: 10 min   **Cooking time:** 8 hrs   **Servings:** 4

Ingredients:

- 1-pound boneless pork butt roast
- Pink Himalayan salt
- Freshly ground black pepper
- 1 tablespoon smoked paprika or Liquid Smoke
- 1/2 cup of water
- 1/2 head cabbage, chopped

Directions:

1. With the crock insert in place, preheat the slow cooker to low.
2. Generously season the pork roast with pink Himalayan salt, pepper, and smoked paprika.
3. Place the pork roast in the slow-cooker insert, and add the water.
4. Cover and cook on low for 7 hours.
5. Transfer the cooked pork roast to a plate. Put the chopped cabbage in the bottom of the slow cooker, and put the pork roast back in on the cabbage.
6. Cover and cook the cabbage and pork roast for 1 hour.
7. Remove the pork roast from the slow cooker and place it on a baking sheet. Use two forks to shred the pork.
8. Serve the shredded pork hot with the cooked cabbage.
9. Reserve the liquid from the slow cooker to remoisten the pork and cabbage when reheating leftovers.

Nutrition:
Calories: 451 kcal   **Fat:** 19.3 g   **Fiber:** 11.2 g   **Carbohydrates:** 2.1 g   **Protein:** 14.2 g

PORK CHOPS IN BLUE CHEESE SAUCE

Prep Time: 5 min   **Cooking time:** 10 min   **Servings:** 2

Ingredients:

- 2 boneless pork chops
- Pink Himalayan salt
- Freshly ground black pepper
- 2 tablespoons butter
- 1/3 cup blue cheese crumbles
- 1/3 cup heavy (whipping) cream
- 1/3 cup sour cream

Directions:

1. Dry the pork chops and season with pink Himalayan salt and pepper.
2. In a medium skillet over medium heat, melt the butter. When the butter melts and is very hot, add the pork chops and sear on each side for 3 minutes.
3. The pork chops must be transferred to a plate and let rest for 3 to 5 minutes.
4. In a preheated pan, melt the blue cheese crumbles, frequently stirring so they don't burn.
5. Add the cream and the sour cream to the pan with the blue cheese. Let simmer for a few minutes, stirring occasionally.
6. For an extra kick of flavor in the sauce, pour the pork-chop pan juice into the cheese mixture and stir. Let simmer while the pork chops are resting.
7. Put the pork chops on two plates, pour the blue cheese sauce over the top of each, and serve.

Nutrition:
Calories: 434 kcal   **Fat:** 14.1 g   **Fiber:** 11.3 g   **Carbohydrates:** 3.1 g   **Protein:** 17.5 g

COCONUT AND LIME STEAK

 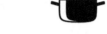

Prep Time: 25 min   **Cooking time:** 15 min   **Servings:** 4

Ingredients:

- 2 pounds steak, grass-fed
- 1 tablespoon minced garlic
- 1 lime, zested
- 1 teaspoon ginger, grated
- 3/4 teaspoon sea salt
- 1 teaspoon red pepper flakes
- 2 tablespoons lime juice
- 1/2 cup coconut oil, melted

Directions:

1. Take a large bowl and add garlic, ginger, salt, red pepper flakes, lime juice, zest, pour in oil, and whisk until combined.
2. Add the steaks, toss until well coated, and marinate at room temperature for 20 minutes.
3. After 20 minutes, take a large skillet pan, place it over medium-high heat, and when hot, add steaks (cut steaks in half if they don't fit into the pan).
4. Cook the steaks and then transfer them to a cutting board.
5. Let steaks cool for 5 minutes, then slice across the grain and serve.

Nutrition:
Calories: 512 kcal   **Fat:** 17.9 g   **Fiber:** 12.5 g   **Carbohydrates:** 4.9 g   **Protein:** 19.9 g

BEEF AND VEGETABLE SKILLET

Prep Time: 5 min   **Cooking time:** 15 min   **Servings:** 2

Ingredients:

- 3 oz spinach, chopped
- 1/2 pound ground beef
- 2 slices of bacon, diced
- 2 oz chopped asparagus
- Seasoning:
- 3 tbsp. coconut oil
- 2 tsp. dried thyme
- 2/3 tsp. salt
- 1/2 tsp. ground black pepper

Directions:

1. Take a skillet pan, place it over medium heat, add oil and when hot, add beef and bacon and cook for 5 to 7 minutes until slightly browned.
2. Then add asparagus and spinach, sprinkle with thyme, stir well and cook for 7 to 10 minutes until thoroughly cooked.
3. Season skillet with salt and black pepper and serve.

Nutrition:
Calories: 332 kcal   **Fat:** 18.4 g   **Fiber:** 9.4 g   **Carbohydrates:** 3.8 g   **Protein:** 14.1 g

BEEF TACO SALAD

 Prep Time: 10 min

 Cooking time: 10 min

 Servings: 2

Ingredients:

- 1-pound ground beef (80/20)
- 1/4 teaspoon pink Himalayan sea salt
- 1/4 teaspoon freshly ground black pepper
- 1/4 cup mayonnaise
- 2 tablespoons sugar-free ketchup
- 2 tablespoons yellow mustard
- 1 tablespoon dill relish
- 1 (8-ounce) bag shredded lettuce
- 1/2 cup sliced red onion
- 1/2 cup chopped ripe tomato
- 1 dill pickle, sliced
- 1/4 cup shredded cheddar cheese

Directions:

1. In a medium sauté pan or skillet, brown the ground beef, stirring, for 7 to 10 minutes. Season with the salt and pepper, then drain the meat, if desired.
2. In a small bowl, combine the mayonnaise, ketchup, mustard, and relish.
3. Fill a large bowl with the shredded lettuce. Top with the beef, red onion, tomato, dill pickle, and cheese. Put dressing, serve.

Nutrition:
Calories: 398 kcal **Fat:** 15.1 g **Fiber:** 12.9 g **Carbohydrates:** 3.1 g **Protein:** 14.8 g

BEEF CHILI

 Prep Time: 10 min

 Cooking time: 50 min

 Servings: 4

Ingredients:

- 1/2 green bell pepper, cored, seeded, and chopped
- 1/2 medium onion, chopped
- 2 tablespoons extra-virgin olive oil
- 1 tablespoon minced garlic
- 1-pound ground beef (80/20)
- 1 (14-ounce) can crushed tomatoes
- 1 cup beef broth
- 1 tablespoon ground cumin
- 1 tablespoon chili powder
- 2 teaspoons paprika
- 1 teaspoon pink Himalayan sea salt
- 1/4 teaspoon cayenne pepper

Directions:

1. In a medium pot, combine the bell pepper, onion, and olive oil. Cook over medium heat for 8 to 10 minutes until the onion, is translucent.
2. Add the garlic and sauté.
3. Add the ground beef and cook for 7 to 10 minutes, until browned.
4. Add the tomatoes, broth, cumin, chili powder, paprika, salt, and cayenne. Stir to combine.
5. Simmer the chili for 30 minutes, until the flavors come together, then enjoy.

Nutrition:
Calories: 376 kcal **Fat:** 18.4 g **Fiber:** 12 g **Carbohydrates:** 3.2 g **Protein:** 15.1 g

EGG ROLL BOWLS

 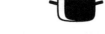

Prep Time: 10 min **Cooking time:** 30 min **Servings:** 4

Ingredients:

- 1 tbsp. vegetable oil
- 1 clove garlic, minced
- 1 tbsp. minced fresh ginger
- 1 lb. ground pork
- 1 tbsp. sesame oil
- 1/2 onion, thinly sliced
- 1 c. shredded carrot
- 1/4 green cabbage, thinly sliced
- 1/4 c. soy sauce
- 1 tbsp. Sriracha
- 1 green onion, thinly sliced
- 1 tbsp. sesame seeds

Directions:

1. Heat oil.
2. Put garlic and ginger and cook until fragrant, about 1 to 2 minutes.
3. Put pork and cook until no pink remains.
4. Push pork to the side and add sesame oil.
5. Put onion, carrot, and cabbage. Stir to combine with meat.
6. Then put soy sauce and Sriracha.
7. Stir and cook until cabbage is tender, about 6 to 8 minutes.
8. Move and mixture to a serving dish
9. Garnish with sesame seeds and the green onions.

Nutrition:
Calories: 321 kcal **Fat:** 15 g **Fiber:** 9.5 g **Carbohydrates:** 5.1 g **Protein:** 7.4 g

PHILLY CHEESE STEAK WRAPS

Prep Time: 10 min   **Cooking time:** 20 min   **Servings:** 4

Ingredients:

- 2 tbsp. vegetable oil, divided
- 1 large onion, thinly sliced
- 2 large bell peppers, thinly sliced
- 1 tsp. dried oregano
- Kosher salt
- Freshly ground black pepper
- 1 lb. skirt steak, thinly sliced
- 1 c. shredded provolone
- 8 large butterhead lettuce leaves
- 2 tbsp. freshly chopped parsley

Directions:

1. Heat 1 tbsp. oil and put chopped onion and sliced bell peppers and sprinkle with oregano, salt, and pepper.
2. Cook, often stirring, until the onion and pepper are tender, about 3-5 minutes.
3. Transfer the cooked peppers and onions to a plate and add the remaining oil in the skillet.
4. Put the steak in the skillet and spread a single layer, season with salt and pepper.
5. Sear until the steak is seared on one side, about 2-3 minutes.
6. Flip and sear on the second side until cooked through, about 2-3 minutes more for medium.
7. Put the cooked and pepper back to skillet and mix to combine.
8. Sprinkle the cheese over onions and steak.
9. Cover the steak skillet with a lid and cook until the cheese has melted, turn off the heat.
10. Lay the lettuce leaves on a serving platter.
11. Top with steak mixture on each piece of lettuce.
12. Garnish with parsley and serve warm.

Nutrition:
Calories: 375 kcal   **Fat:** 15.1 g   **Fiber:** 12.9 g   **Carbohydrates:** 4.3 g   **Protein:** 17.5 g

SWEDISH MEATBALLS

Prep Time: 15 min   **Cooking time:** 20 min   **Servings:** 4

Ingredients:

- Swedish Meatballs
- 1-pound ground beef
- 1 tbsp. dried parsley
- 1/4 tsp. allspice
- 1/4 tsp. nutmeg
- 1/2 tsp. garlic powder
- Salt and pepper, to taste
- 1/4 onion, diced
- 2 tbsp. butter
- Beef Gravy
- 4 tbsp. butter
- 1 1/2 cups beef stock
- 1/2 cup heavy whipping cream
- 1/2 cup sour cream
- 2 tbsp. Worcestershire sauce
- 1/2 tbsp. Dijon mustard
- Salt and pepper, to taste

Directions:

1. Combine the ground beef, dried parsley, allspice, nutmeg, garlic powder, salt, pepper, and onion in a large mixing bowl.
2. Mix the mixture with your hands and shape into 20 even-sized balls.
3. In a skillet, melt the butter and cook the meatball in batches.
4. Cook the meatball on all sides until golden browned and baste with the butter, set aside.
5. Heat the butter in a pan for the gravy, scrape up the browned bits from the bottom.
6. Add the beef stock, whipping cream, sour cream, Worcestershire sauce, Dijon mustard, salt, and pepper in the pan, then whisk together.
7. Mix the xanthan gum with a ladleful of sauce and
8. Pour in the gravy, stirring continuously.
9. Stir in the meatballs back to the gravy pan, coating the meatballs with the gravy.
10. Simmer for another 15 minutes until cooked through. Serve mashed cauliflower.

Nutrition:
Calories: 378 kcal   **Fat:** 10.4 g   **Fiber:** 5.3 g   **Carbohydrates:** 3.1 g   **Protein:** 17.5 g

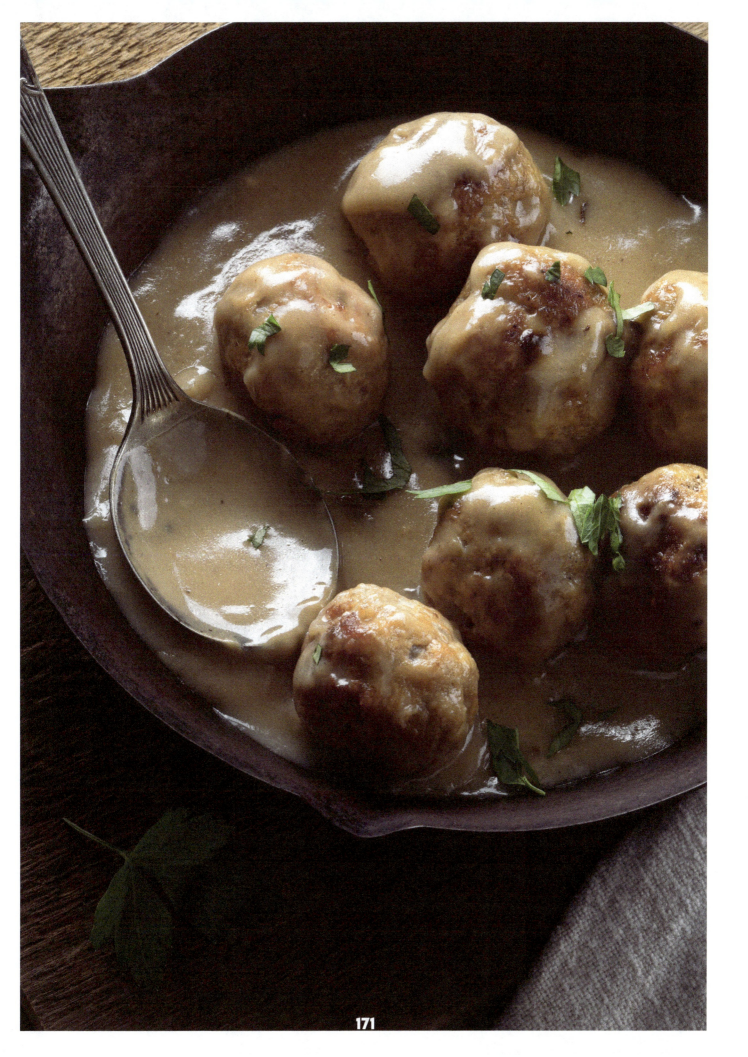

GROUND BEEF STROGANOFF

 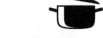

Prep Time: 10 min **Cooking time:** 15 min **Servings:** 4

Ingredients:

- 2 tbsp. butter
- 1 clove minced garlic
- 1 pound 80% lean ground beef
- Salt and pepper, to taste
- 10 oz(228g) sliced mushrooms
- 2 tbsp. water
- 1 cup sour cream
- 1 tbsp. fresh lemon juice
- 1 tbsp. fresh chopped parsley

Directions:

1. The butter must be added to a pan. When the butter has melted and stops foaming, add the minced garlic to the skillet.
2. Cook the garlic until fragrant, then mix in the ground beef—season with salt and pepper.
3. Cook the ground beef until no longer pink; break up the grounds with a wooden spoon.
4. Add the water and mushrooms to the pan and cook over medium heat.
5. Cook until the liquid has reduced halfway, and the mushrooms are tender. Set the cooked mushrooms aside.
6. Reduce the heat, then whisk the sour cream and paprika into the skillet.
7. Stir in the cooked beef and mushrooms into the pan and combine. Stir in the lemon juice and parsley.

Nutrition:
Calories: 380 kcal **Fat:** 15.1 g **Fiber:** 3.6 g **Carbohydrates:** 12.3 g **Protein:** 15.4 g

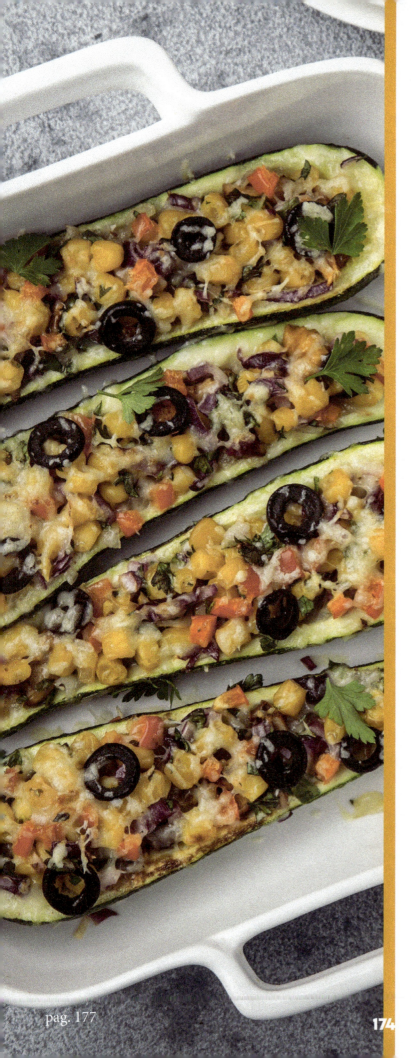

15

VEGETABLES RECIPES

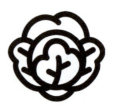

VEGETARIAN CHILI WITH AVOCADO CREAM

Prep Time: 15 min   **Cooking time:** 25 min   **Servings:** 8

Ingredients:

- 2 tablespoons olive oil
- 1/2 onion, finely chopped
- 1 tablespoon minced garlic
- 2 jalapeño peppers, chopped
- 1 red bell pepper, diced
- 1 teaspoon ground cumin
- 2 tablespoons chili powder
- 2 cups pecans, chopped
- 4 cups canned diced tomatoes and their juice

Topping:

- 1 cup sour cream
- 1 avocado, diced
- 2 tablespoons fresh cilantro, chopped

Directions:

1. Heat olive oil.
2. Toss in the onion, garlic, jalapeño peppers, and red bell pepper, then sauté for about 4 minutes until tender.
3. Put in the chili powder and cumin and stir for 30 seconds.
4. Fold in the pecans, tomatoes, and their juice, then bring to a boil.
5. Simmer uncovered for about 20 minutes to infuse the flavors, stirring occasionally.
6. Remove from the heat to eight bowls.
7. Evenly top each bowl of chili with the sour cream, diced avocado, and fresh cilantro.

Nutrition:
Calories: 318 kcal   **Fat:** 14.4 g   **Fiber:** 17.5 g   **Carbohydrates:** 9.5 g   **Protein:** 14 g

STUFFED ZUCCHINI

Prep Time: 20 min   **Cooking time:** 20 min   **Servings:** 4

Ingredients:

- 4 medium zucchinis, halved lengthwise
- 1 cup red bell pepper, seeded and minced
- 1/2 cup Kalamata olives, pitted and minced
- 1/2 cup fresh tomatoes, minced
- 1 teaspoon garlic, minced
- 1 tablespoon dried oregano, crushed
- Salt and ground black pepper, as required
- 1/2 cup feta cheese, crumbled

Directions:

1. Grease a large baking sheet.
2. With a melon baller, scoop out the flesh of each zucchini half. Discard the flesh.
3. In a bowl, mix the bell pepper, olives, tomatoes, garlic, oregano, salt, and black pepper.
4. Stuff each zucchini half with the veggie mixture evenly.
5. Arrange zucchini halves onto the prepared baking sheet and bake for about 15 minutes.
6. Now, set the oven to broiler on high.
7. Top each zucchini half with feta cheese and broil for about 3 minutes.
8. Serve hot.

Nutrition:
Calories: 314 kcal **Fat:** 12.4 g **Fiber:** 9.4 g **Carbohydrates:** 4.1 g **Protein:** 7.4 g

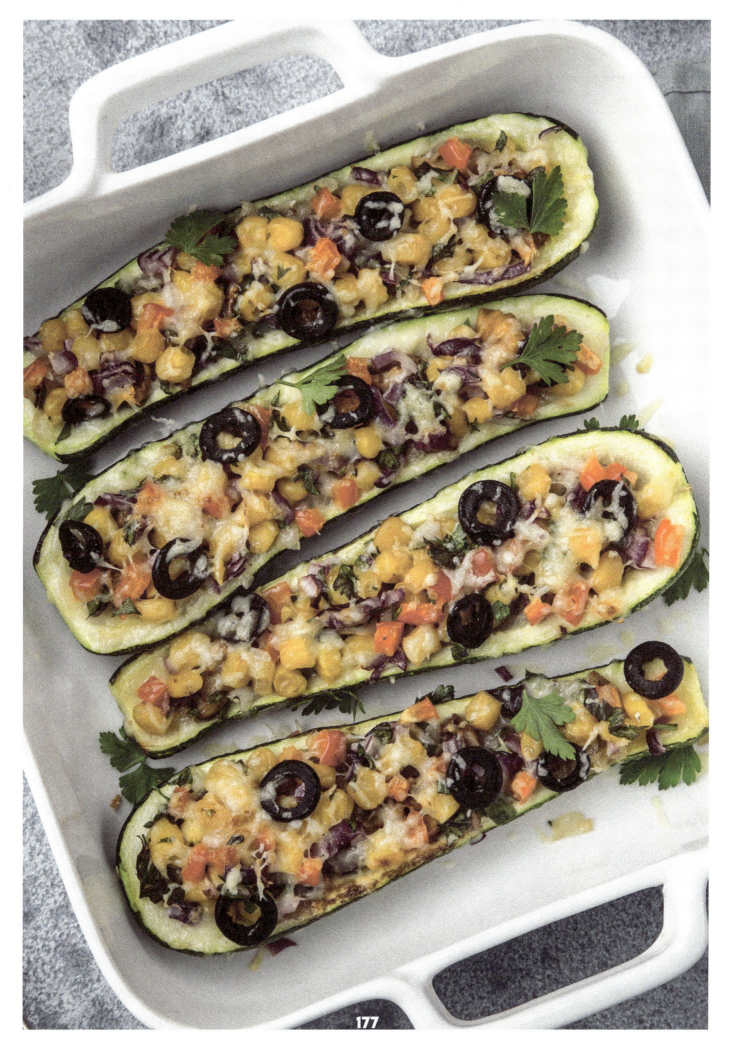

CREAMY ZOODLES

Prep Time: 15 min **Cooking time:** 10 min **Servings:** 4

Ingredients:

- 1 1/4 cups heavy whipping cream
- 1/4 cup mayonnaise
- Salt and ground black pepper, as required
- 30 ounces zucchini, spiralized with blade C
- 3 ounces Parmesan cheese, grated
- 2 tablespoons fresh mint leaves
- 2 tablespoons butter, melted

Directions:

1. The heavy cream must be added to a pan then bring to a boil.
2. Lower the heat to low and cook until reduced in half.
3. Put in the pepper, mayo, and salt; cook until mixture is warm enough.
4. Add the zucchini noodles and gently stir to combine.
5. Stir in the Parmesan cheese.
6. Divide the zucchini noodles onto four serving plates and immediately drizzle with the melted butter.
7. Serve immediately.

Nutrition:
Calories: 241 kcal **Fat:** 11.4 g **Fiber:** 7.5 g **Carbohydrates:** 3.1 g **Protein:** 5.1 g

CHERRY TOMATO GRATIN

Prep Time: 15 min   **Cooking time:** 20 min   **Servings:** 4

Ingredients:

- 2 tablespoons olive oil,
- 1/2 cup cherry tomatoes halved
- 1/2 cup mayonnaise, Keto-friendly
- 1/2 cup vegan Mozzarella cheese, cut into pieces
- 1 ounce (28 g) vegan Parmesan cheese, shredded
- 1 tablespoon basil pesto
- Pepper and salt
- 1 cup watercress

Directions:

1. Let the oven heat up to 400F. Grease a baking pan with olive oil.
2. Combine the cherry tomatoes, mayo, vegan Mozzarella cheese, 1/2 ounce (14 g) of Parmesan cheese, basil pesto, salt, and black pepper baking pan.
3. Scatter with the remaining Parmesan.
4. Baking time: 20 minutes
5. Remove them from the oven and divide among four plates. Top with watercress and olive oil, and slice to serve.

Nutrition:
Calories: 254 kcal   **Fat:** 12.1 g   **Fiber:** 9.3 g   **Carbohydrates:** 11.1 g   **Protein:** 9.5 g

BLACK BEAN VEGGIE BURGER

 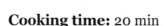

Prep Time: 15 min   **Cooking time:** 20 min   **Servings:** 2

Ingredients:

- 1/2 onion (chopped small)
- 1 (14-ounce) can of black beans (well-drained)
- 2 slices of bread (crumbled)
- 1/2 teaspoon of seasoned salt
- 1 teaspoon of garlic powder
- 1 teaspoon of onion powder
- 1/2 cup of almond flour
- Dash salt (to taste)
- Dash pepper (to taste)
- Oil for frying (divide

Directions:

1. Combine onions and sauté and pour it in the small frying pan. Fry them until they are soft. This process usually takes between 3 and 5 minutes.
2. Get a large bowl. Mash the black beans inside it. Ensure that the beans are almost smooth.
3. Sauté your onions and crumble the bread.
4. In the bowl, add the sautéed onions, mashed black beans, crumbled bread, seasoned salt, garlic powder, and onion powder. Ensure you mix to combine well.
5. Add some flour to the ingredients by adding a teaspoon per time. Stir everything together until it is well combined.
6. While mixing, make sure that it is very thick.
7. To achieve this, you may want to use your hand to work your flour well.
8. Make the mixed black beans into patties.
9. Ensure that each of the patties is approximately 1/2 inch thick.
10. The best way to do this is to make a ball with the black beans.
11. After doing this, flatten the ball gently. Place your frying pan on medium-low heat. Add some oil.
12. Fry your black bean patties in the frying pan until it is slightly firm and lightly browned on each side. This usually takes about 3 minutes.
13. Ensure you adjust the
14. head well because if the pan is too hot, the bean burgers will be brown in the middle and will not be well cooked in the middle.
15. To serve, assemble your veggie burgers and enjoy it with all the fixings.
16. You can also serve get a plate, serve them with a little ketchup or hot sauce.
17. To increase the nutrition of the meal, you can add a nice green salad.

Nutrition:
Calories: 376 kcal   **Fat:** 15.1 g   **Fiber:** 12.9 g   **Carbohydrates:** 9.4 g   **Protein:** 11.6 g

KETO RED CURRY

Prep Time: 20 min   **Cooking time:** 15/20 min   **Servings:** 6

Ingredients:

- 1 cup broccoli florets
- 1 large handful of fresh spinach
- 4 Tbsp. coconut oil
- 1/4 medium onion
- 1 tsp. garlic, minced
- 1 tsp. fresh ginger, peeled and minced
- 2 tsp. soy sauce
- 1 Tbsp. red curry paste
- 1/2 cup coconut cream

Directions:

1. Add half the coconut oil to a saucepan and heat over medium-high heat.
2. When the oil is hot, put in the onion to the pan and sauté for 3-4 minutes, until it is semi-translucent.
3. Sauté garlic, stirring, just until fragrant, about 30 seconds.
4. Lower the heat to medium-low and add broccoli florets. Sauté, stirring, for about 1-2 minutes.
5. Now, add the red curry paste. Sauté until the paste is fragrant, then mix everything.
6. Add the spinach on top of the vegetable mixture. When the spinach begins to wilt, add the coconut cream and stir.
7. Add the rest of the coconut oil, the soy sauce, and the minced ginger. Bring to a simmer for 5-10 minutes.
8. Serve hot.

Nutrition:
Calories: 265 kcal   **Fat:** 7.1 g   **Fiber:** 6.9 g   **Carbohydrates:** 2.1 g   **Protein:** 4.4 g

SWEET-AND-SOUR TEMPEH

 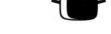

Prep Time: 10 min   **Cooking time:** 25 min   **Servings:** 4

Ingredients:

- Tempeh
- 1 package of tempeh
- 3/4 cup of vegetable broth
- 2 tablespoons of soy sauce
- 2 tablespoons olive oil
- Sauce
- 1 can of pineapple juice
- 2 tablespoons of brown sugar
- 1/4 cup of white vinegar
- 1 tablespoon of cornstarch
- 1 red bell pepper
- 1 chopped white onion

Directions:

1. Place a skillet on high heat. Pour in the vegetable broth and tempeh in it.
2. Add the soy sauce to the tempeh. Let it cook until it softens. This usually takes 10 minutes.
3. When it is well cooked, remove the tempeh and keep the liquid. We are going to use it for the sauce.
4. Put the tempeh in another skillet placed on medium heat.
5. Sauté it with olive oil and cook until the tempeh is browned. This should take 3 minutes.
6. Place a pot of the reserved liquid from the cooked tempeh on medium heat.
7. Add the pineapple juice, vinegar, brown sugar, and cornstarch. Stir everything together until it's well combined.
8. Let it simmer for 5 minutes.
9. Add the onion and pepper to the sauce.
10. Stir in until the sauce is thick.
11. Reduce the heat, add the cooked tempeh and pineapple chunks to the sauce. Leave it to simmer together.
12. Remove from heat and serve with any grain food of your choice.

Nutrition:
Calories: 312 kcal   **Fat:** 10 g   **Fiber:** 4.1 g   **Carbohydrates:** 2.1 g   **Protein:** 5.2 g

MEXICAN CASSEROLE WITH BLACK BEANS

Prep Time: 20 min   **Cooking time:** 20 min   **Servings:** 6

Ingredients:

- 2 cups of minced garlic cloves
- 2 cups of Monterey Jack and cheddar
- 3/4 cup of salsa
- 1 1/2 cups chopped red pepper
- 2 teaspoons ground cumin
- 2 cans black beans
- 12 corn tortillas
- 3 chopped tomatoes
- 1/2 cup of sliced black olives
- 2 cups of chopped onion

Directions:

1. Let the oven heat to 350F.
2. Place a large pot over medium heat.
3. Pour the onion, garlic, pepper, cumin, salsa, and black beans in the pot — Cook the ingredients for 3 minutes, stirring frequently.
4. Arrange the tortillas in the baking dish.
5. Ensure they are well spaced and even overlapping the dish if necessary.
6. Spread half of the bean's mixture on the tortillas. Sprinkle with the cheddar.
7. Repeat the process across the tortillas until everything is well stuffed.
8. Cover the baking dish with foil paper and place in the oven.
9. Bake it for 15 minutes. Remove from the oven to cool down a bit.
10. Garnish the casserole with olives and tomatoes

Nutrition:
Calories: 325 kcal   **Fat:** 9.4 g   **Fiber:** 11.2 g   **Carbohydrates:** 3.1 g   **Protein:** 12.6 g

VEGGIE GREEK MOUSSAKA

Prep Time: 20 min   **Cooking time:** 30 min   **Servings:** 6

Ingredients:

- 2 large eggplants, cut into strips
- 1 cup diced celery
- 1 cup diced carrots
- 1 small white onion, chopped
- 2 eggs
- 1 tsp. olive oil
- 3 cups grated Parmesan
- 1 cup ricotta cheese
- 3 cloves garlic, minced
- 2 tsp. Italian seasoning blend
- Salt to taste

Sauce:

- 1 1/2 cups heavy cream
- 1/4 cup butter, melted
- 1 cup grated mozzarella cheese
- 2 tsp. Italian seasoning
- 3/4 cup almond flour

Directions:

1. Preheat the oven to 350°F.
2. Lay the eggplant strips, sprinkle with salt, and let sit there to exude liquid. Heat olive oil heat and sauté the onion, celery, garlic, and carrots for 5 minutes.
3. Mix the eggs, 1 cup of Parmesan cheese, ricotta cheese, and salt in a bowl; set aside.
4. Pour the heavy cream in a pot and bring to heat over a medium fire while continually stirring.
5. Stir in the remaining Parmesan cheese and one teaspoon of Italian seasoning. Turn the heat off and set aside.
6. To lay the moussaka, spread a small amount of the sauce at the bottom of the baking dish.
7. Pat dry the eggplant strips and make a single layer on the sauce.
8. A layer of ricotta cheese must be spread on the eggplants, sprinkle some veggies on it, and repeat everything
9. In a small bowl, evenly mix the melted butter, almond flour, and one teaspoon of Italian seasoning.
10. Spread the top of the moussaka layers with it and sprinkle the top with mozzarella cheese.
11. Bake for 25 minutes until the cheese is slightly burned. Slice the moussaka and serve warm.

Nutrition:
Calories: 398 kcal   **Fat:** 15.1 g   **Fiber:** 11.3 g   **Carbohydrates:** 3.1 g   **Protein:** 5.9 g

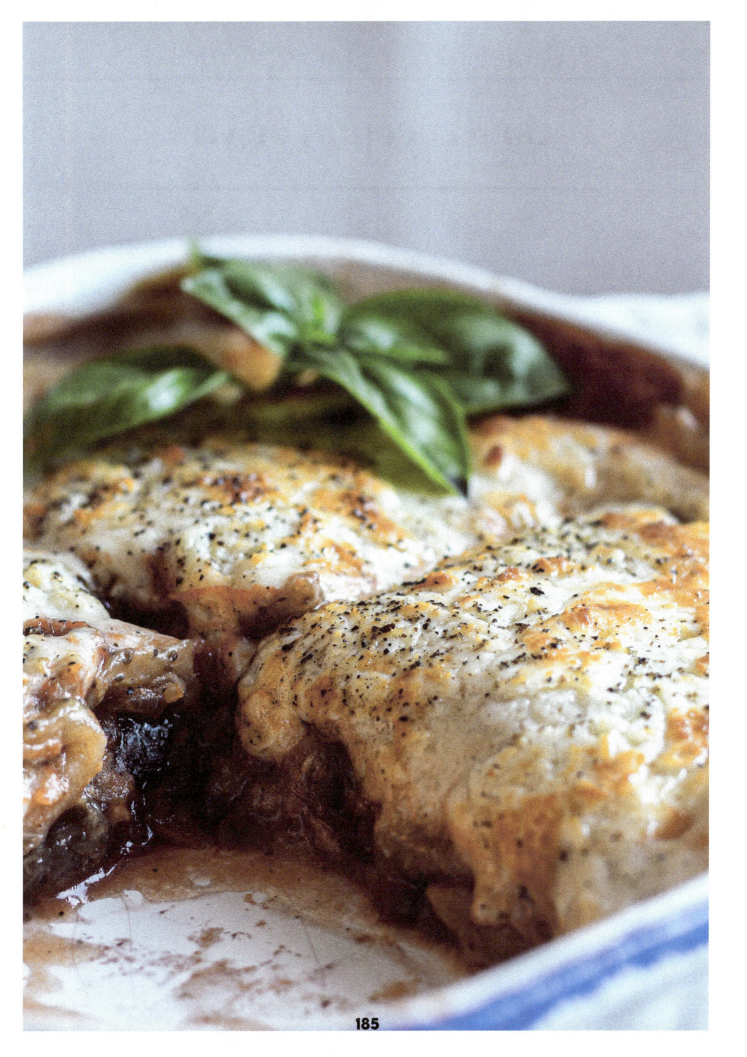

BAKED ZUCCHINI GRATIN

Prep Time: 25 min   **Cooking time:** 30 min   **Servings:** 2

Ingredients:

- 1 large zucchini, cut into 1/4-inch-thick slices
- Pink Himalayan salt
- 1-ounce Brie cheese, rind trimmed off
- 1 tablespoon butter
- Freshly ground black pepper
- 1/3 cup shredded Gruyere cheese
- 1/4 cup crushed pork rinds

Directions:

1. Preheat the oven to 400°F.
2. When the zucchini has been "weeping" for about 30 minutes, in a small saucepan over medium-low heat, heat the Brie and butter, occasionally stirring, until the cheese has melted.
3. The mixture is thoroughly combined for about 2 minutes.
4. Arrange the zucchini in an 8-inch baking dish, so the zucchini slices are overlapping a bit.
5. Season with pepper.
6. Pour the Brie mixture over the zucchini, and top with the shredded Gruyere cheese.
7. Sprinkle the crushed pork rinds over the top.
8. Bake for about 25 minutes, until the dish is bubbling and the top is nicely browned, and serve.

Nutrition:
Calories: 324 kcal   **Fat:** 11.5 g   **Fiber:** 5.1 g   **Carbohydrates:** 2.2 g   **Protein:** 5.1 g

GOUDA CAULIFLOWER CASSEROLE

Prep Time: 15 min   **Cooking time:** 15 min   **Servings:** 4

Ingredients:

- 2 heads cauliflower, cut into florets
- 1/3 cup butter, cubed
- 2 tbsp. melted butter
- 1 white onion, chopped
- Salt and black pepper to taste
- 1/4 almond milk
- 1/2 cup almond flour
- 1 1/2 cups grated gouda cheese

Directions:

1. Preheat oven to 350°F and put the cauliflower florets in a large microwave-safe bowl.
2. Sprinkle with a bit of water, and steam in the microwave for 4 to 5 minutes.
3. Melt the 1/3 cup of butter in a saucepan over medium heat and sauté the onion for 3 minutes.
4. Add the cauliflower, season with salt and black pepper, and mix in almond milk. Simmer for 3 minutes.
5. Mix the remaining melted butter with almond flour.
6. Stir into the cauliflower as well as half of the cheese. Sprinkle the top with the remaining cheese and bake for 10 minutes until the cheese has melted and golden brown.
7. Plate the bake and serve with salad.

Nutrition:
Calories: 349 kcal   **Fat:** 9.4 g   **Fiber:** 12.1 g   **Carbohydrates:** 4.1 g   **Protein:** 10 g

SPINACH AND ZUCCHINI LASAGNA

Prep Time: 15 min　　**Cooking time:** 30 min　　**Servings:** 4

Ingredients:

- 2 zucchinis, sliced
- Salt and black pepper to taste
- 2 cups ricotta cheese
- 2 cups shredded mozzarella cheese
- 3 cups tomato sauce
- 1 cup baby spinach

Directions:

1. Let the oven heat to 375 and grease a baking dish with cooking spray.
2. Put the zucchini slices in a colander and sprinkle with salt.
3. Let sit and drain liquid for 5 minutes and pat dry with paper towels.
4. Mix the ricotta, mozzarella cheese, salt, and black pepper to evenly combine and spread 1/4 cup of the mixture in the bottom of the baking dish.
5. Layer 1/3 of the zucchini slices on top spread 1 cup of tomato sauce over, and scatter a 1/3 cup of spinach on top. Repeat process.
6. Grease one end of foil with cooking spray and cover the baking dish with the foil.
7. Let it bake for about 35 minutes. And bake further for 5 to 10 minutes or until the cheese has a nice golden-brown color.
8. Remove the dish, sit for 5 minutes, make slices of the lasagna, and serve warm.

Nutrition:
Calories: 376 kcal　**Fat:** 14.1 g　**Fiber:** 11.3 g　**Carbohydrates:** 2.1 g　**Protein:** 9.5 g

LEMON CAULIFLOWER "COUSCOUS" WITH HALLOUMI

Prep Time: 5 min   **Cooking time:** 15 min   **Servings:** 2

Ingredients:

- 4 oz halloumi, sliced
- 1 cauliflower head, cut into small florets
- 1/4 cup chopped cilantro
- 1/4 cup chopped parsley
- 1/4 cup chopped mint
- 1/2 lemon juiced
- Salt and black pepper to taste
- Sliced avocado to garnish

Directions:

1. Heat the pan and add oil
2. Add the halloumi and fry on both sides until golden brown, set aside. Turn the heat off.
3. Next, pour the cauliflower florets in a food processor and pulse until it crumbles and resembles couscous.
4. Transfer to a bowl and steam in the microwave for 2 minutes.
5. They should be slightly cooked but crunchy.
6. Stir in the cilantro, parsley, mint, lemon juice, salt, and black pepper.
7. Garnish the couscous with avocado slices and serve with grilled halloumi and vegetable sauce.

Nutrition:
Calories: 312 kcal   **Fat:** 9.4 g   **Fiber:** 11.9 g   **Carbohydrates:** 1.2 g   **Protein:** 8.5 g

SPICY CAULIFLOWER STEAKS WITH STEAMED GREEN BEANS

Prep Time: 15 min

Cooking time: 20 min

Servings: 4

Ingredients:

- 2 heads cauliflower, sliced lengthwise into 'steaks.'
- 1/4 cup olive oil
- 1/4 cup chili sauce
- 2 tsp. erythritol
- Salt and black pepper to taste
- 2 shallots, diced
- 1 bunch green beans, trimmed
- 2 tbsp. fresh lemon juice
- 1 cup of water
- Dried parsley to garnish

Directions:

1. In a bowl or container, mix the olive oil, chili sauce, and erythritol.
2. Brush the cauliflower with the mixture. Grill for 6 minutes. Flip the cauliflower, cook further for 6 minutes.
3. Let the water boil, place the green beans in a sieve, and set over the steam from the boiling water.
4. Cover with a clean napkin to keep the steam trapped in the sieve.
5. Cook for 6 minutes.
6. After, remove to a bowl and toss with lemon juice.
7. Remove the grilled caulis to a plate; sprinkle with salt, pepper, shallots, and parsley. Serve with the steamed green beans.

Nutrition:
Calories: 329 kcal   **Fat:** 10.4 g   **Fiber:** 3.1 g   **Carbohydrates:** 4.2 g   **Protein:** 8.4 g

CHEESY CAULIFLOWER FALAFEL

Prep Time: 20 min   **Cooking time:** 15 min   **Servings:** 4

Ingredients:

- 1 head cauliflower, cut into florets
- 1/3 cup silvered ground almonds
- 2 tbsp. cheddar cheese, shredded
- 1/2 tsp. mixed spice
- Salt and chili pepper to taste
- 3 tbsp. coconut flour
- 3 fresh eggs
- 4 tbsp. ghee

Directions:

1. Blend the florets in a blender until a grain meal consistency is formed.
2. Pour the rice in a bowl, add the ground almonds, mixed spice, salt, cheddar cheese, chili pepper, coconut flour, and mix until evenly combined.
3. Beat the eggs in a bowl until creamy in color and mix with the cauliflower mixture.
4. Shape 1/4 cup each into patties.
5. Melt ghee and fry the patties for 5 minutes on each side to be firm and browned.
6. Remove onto a wire rack to cool, share into serving plates, and top with tahini sauce.

Nutrition:
Calories: 287 kcal   **Fat:** 9.2 g   **Fiber:** 4.1 g   **Carbohydrates:** 3.2 g   **Protein:** 13.2 g

EGGPLANT PIZZA WITH TOFU

Prep Time: 15 min **Cooking time:** 45 min **Servings:** 2

Ingredients:

- 2 eggplants, sliced
- 1/3 cup butter, melted
- 2 garlic cloves, minced
- 1 red onion
- 12 oz tofu, chopped
- 7 oz tomato sauce
- Salt and black pepper to taste
- 1/2 tsp. cinnamon powder
- 1 cup Parmesan cheese, shredded
- 1/4 cup dried oregano

Directions:

1. Let the oven heat to 400F. Lay the eggplant slices in a baking sheet and brush with some butter. Bake in the oven until lightly browned, about 20 minutes.
2. Heat the remaining butter in a skillet; sauté garlic and onion until fragrant and soft, about 3 minutes.
3. Stir in the tofu and cook for 3 minutes. Add the tomato sauce, salt and black pepper. Simmer for 10 minutes.
4. Sprinkle with the Parmesan cheese and oregano. Bake for 10 minutes.

Nutrition:
Calories: 321 kcal **Fat:** 11.3 g **Fiber:** 8.4 g **Carbohydrates:** 4.3 g **Protein:** 10.1 g

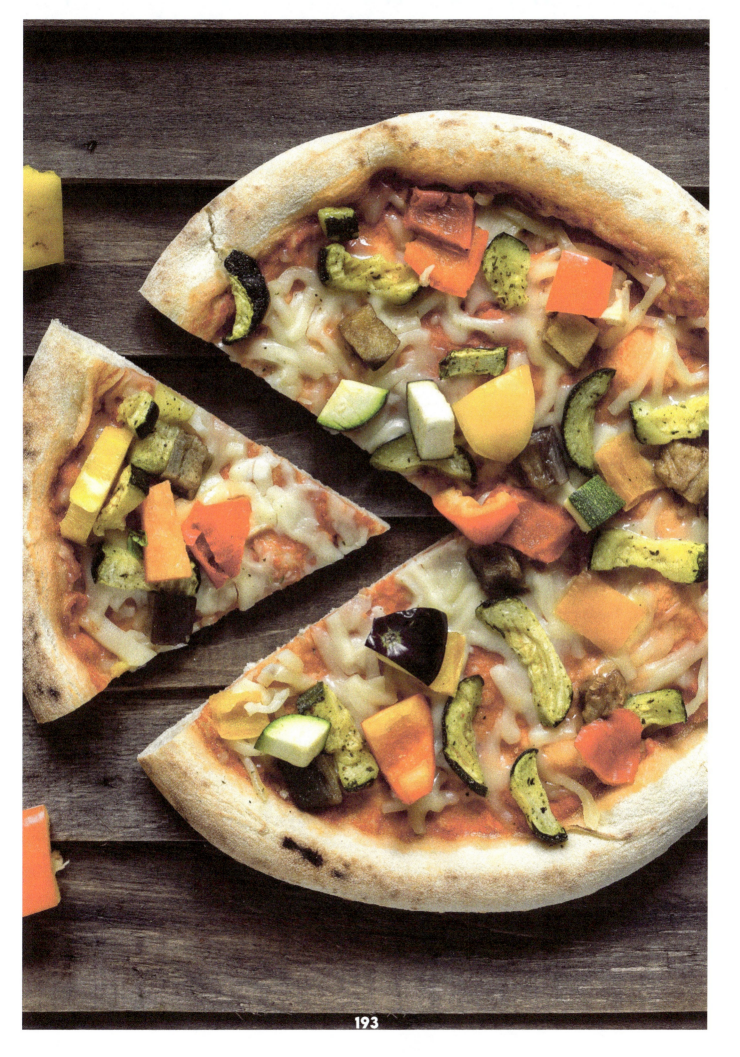

TOFU SESAME SKEWERS WITH WARM KALE SALAD

Prep Time: 2 hrs   **Cooking time:** 25 min   **Servings:** 4

Ingredients:

- 14 oz Firm tofu
- 4 tsp. sesame oil
- 1 lemon, juiced
- 5 tbsp. sugar-free soy sauce
- 3 tsp. garlic powder
- 4 tbsp. coconut flour
- 1/2 cup sesame seeds
- Warm Kale Salad:
- 4 cups chopped kale
- 2 tsp. + 2 tsp. olive oil
- 1 white onion, thinly sliced
- 3 cloves garlic, minced
- 1 cup sliced white mushrooms
- 1 tsp. chopped rosemary
- Salt and black pepper to season
- 1 tbsp. balsamic vinegar

Directions:

1. In a bowl, mix sesame oil, lemon juice, soy sauce, garlic powder, and coconut flour.
2. Wrap the tofu in a paper towel, squeeze out as much liquid from it, and cut it into strips.
3. Stick on the skewers, height-wise.
4. Place onto a plate, pour the soy sauce mixture over, and turn in the sauce to be adequately coated.
5. Heat the griddle pan over high heat.
6. Pour the sesame seeds in a plate and roll the tofu skewers in the seeds for a generous coat.
7. Grill the tofu in the griddle pan to be golden brown on both sides, about 12 minutes.
8. Heat 2 tablespoons of olive oil in a skillet over medium heat and sauté onion to begin browning for 10 minutes with continuous stirring.
9. Add the remaining olive oil and mushrooms.
10. Continue cooking for 10 minutes. Add garlic, rosemary, salt, pepper, and balsamic vinegar.
11. Cook for 1 minute.
12. Put the kale in a salad bowl; when the onion mixture is ready, pour it on the kale and toss well.
13. Serve the tofu skewers with the warm kale salad and a peanut butter dipping sauce.

Nutrition:
Calories: 276 kcal   **Fat:** 11.9 g   **Fiber:** 9.4 g   **Carbohydrates:** 21 g   **Protein:** 10.3 g

BRUSSEL SPROUTS WITH SPICED HALLOUMI

Prep Time: 20 min   **Cooking time:** 30min   **Servings:** 2

Ingredients:

- 10 oz halloumi cheese, sliced
- 1 tbsp. coconut oil
- 1/2 cup unsweetened coconut, shredded
- 1 tsp. chili powder
- 1/2 tsp. onion powder
- 1/2 pound Brussels sprouts, shredded
- 4 oz butter
- Salt and black pepper to taste
- Lemon wedges for serving

Directions:

1. In a bowl, mix the shredded coconut, chili powder, salt, coconut oil, and onion powder.
2. Then, toss the halloumi slices in the spice mixture.
3. The grill pan must be heated then cook the coated halloumi cheese for 2-3 minutes.
4. Transfer to a plate to keep warm.
5. The half butter must be melted in a pan, add, and sauté the Brussels sprouts until slightly caramelized.
6. Then, season with salt and black pepper.
7. Dish the Brussels sprouts into serving plates with the halloumi cheese and lemon wedges.
8. Melt left butter and drizzle over the Brussels sprouts and halloumi cheese. Serve.

Nutrition:
Calories: 276 kcal   **Fat:** 9.5 g   **Fiber:** 9.1 g   **Carbohydrates:** 4.1 g   **Protein:** 5.4 g

CHEESY STUFFED PEPPERS

Prep Time: 15 min   **Cooking time:** 40 min   **Servings:** 4

Ingredients:

- 2 tbsp. olive oil
- 4 red bell peppers, halved and seeded
- 1 cup ricotta cheese
- 1/2 cup gorgonzola cheese, crumbled
- 2 cloves garlic, minced
- 1 1/2 cups tomatoes, chopped
- 1 tsp. dried basil
- Salt and black pepper, to taste
- 1/2 tsp. oregano

Directions:

1. Let the oven heat up to 350F.
2. In a bowl, mix garlic, tomatoes, gorgonzola, and ricotta cheeses.
3. Stuff the pepper halves and remove them to the baking dish. Season with oregano, salt, cayenne pepper, black pepper, and basil.
4. Baking Time: 40 minutes

Nutrition:
Calories: 295 kcal   **Fat:** 12.4 g   **Fiber:** 10.1 g   **Carbohydrates:** 5.4 g   **Protein:** 13.2 g

VEGETABLE PATTIES

Prep Time: 15 min **Cooking time:** 20min **Servings:** 4

Ingredients:

- 1 tbsp. olive oil
- 1 onion, chopped
- 1 garlic clove, minced
- 1/2 head cauliflower, grated
- 1 carrot, shredded
- 3 tbsp. coconut flour
- 1/2 cup Gruyere cheese, shredded
- 1/2 cup Parmesan cheese, grated
- 2 eggs, beaten
- 1/2 tsp. dried rosemary
- Salt and black pepper, to taste

Directions:

1. Cook onion and garlic in warm olive oil over medium heat, until soft, for about 3 minutes.
2. Stir in grated cauliflower and carrot and cook for a minute; allow cooling and set aside.
3. To the cooled vegetables, add the rest of the ingredients, form balls from the mixture, then press each ball to form burger patty.
4. Set oven to 400 F and bake the burgers for 20 minutes.
5. Flip and bake for another 10 minutes or until the top become golden brown.

Nutrition:
Calories: 315 kcal **Fat:** 12.1 g **Fiber:** 8.6 g **Carbohydrates:** 3.3 g **Protein:** 5.8 g

PIZZA BIANCA

Prep Time: 10 min   **Cooking time:** 10min   **Servings:** 2

Ingredients:

- 2 tbsp. olive oil
- 4 eggs
- 2 tbsp. water
- 1 jalapeño pepper, diced
- 1/4 cup mozzarella cheese, shredded
- 2 chives, chopped
- 2 cups egg Alfredo sauce
- 1/2 tsp. oregano
- 1/2 cup mushrooms, sliced

Directions:

1. Preheat oven to 360 F.
2. In a bowl, whisk eggs, water, and oregano. Heat the olive oil in a large skillet.
3. The egg mixture must be poured in then let it cook until set, flipping once.
4. Remove and spread the alfredo sauce and jalapeño pepper all over.
5. Top with mozzarella cheese, mushrooms and chives. Let it bake for 10 minutes

Nutrition:
Calories: 314 kcal   **Fat:** 15.6 g   **Fiber:** 10.3 g   **Carbohydrates:** 5.9 g   **Protein:** 10.4 g

GREEK VEGGIE BRIAM

Prep Time: 10 min **Cooking time:** 30 min **Servings:** 4

Ingredients:

- 1/3 cup good-quality olive oil, divided
- 1 onion, thinly sliced
- 1 tablespoon minced garlic
- 3/4 small eggplant, diced
- 2 zucchinis, diced
- 2 cups chopped cauliflower
- 1 red bell pepper, diced
- 2 cups diced tomatoes
- 2 tablespoons chopped fresh parsley
- 2 tablespoons chopped fresh oregano
- Sea salt, for seasoning
- Freshly ground black pepper, for seasoning
- 11/2 cups crumbled feta cheese
- 1/4 cup pumpkin seeds

Directions:

1. Preheat the oven. Set the oven to broil and lightly grease a 9-by-13-inch casserole dish with olive oil.
2. Sauté the aromatics in a medium stockpot over medium heat, warm 3 tablespoons of the olive oil. Add the onion and garlic and sauté until they've softened about 3 minutes.
3. Sauté the vegetables. Stir in the eggplant, cook, stirring occasionally.
4. Add the zucchini, cauliflower, and red bell pepper and cook for 5 minutes.
5. Stir in the tomatoes, parsley, and oregano and cook, stirring it from time to time, until the vegetables are tender, about 10 minutes. Season it with salt and pepper.
6. Broil. Put vegetable mix in the casserole dish and top with the crumbled feta. Broil until the cheese is melted.
7. Serve. Divide the casserole between four plates and top it with the pumpkin seeds. Drizzle with the remaining olive oil.

Nutrition:
Calories: 341 kcal **Fat:** 5.1 g **Fiber:** 11 g **Carbohydrates:** 1.2 g **Protein:** 1.4 g

VEGAN SANDWICH WITH TOFU & LETTUCE SLAW

Prep Time: 15 min   **Cooking time:** 15 min   **Servings:** 2

Ingredients:

- 1/4 pound firm tofu, sliced
- 2 low carb buns
- 1 tbsp. olive oil
- Marinade
- 2 tbsp. olive oil
- Salt and black pepper to taste
- 1 tsp. allspice
- 1/2 tbsp. xylitol
- 1 tsp. thyme, chopped
- 1 habanero pepper, seeded and minced
- 2 green onions, thinly sliced
- 1 garlic clove
- Lettuce slaw
- 1/2 small iceberg lettuce, shredded
- 1/2 carrot, grated
- 1/2 red onion, grated
- 2 tsp. liquid stevia
- 1 tbsp. lemon juice
- 2 tbsp. olive oil
- 1/2 tsp. Dijon mustard
- Salt and black pepper to taste

Directions:

1. Put the tofu slices in a bowl.
2. Blend the marinade ingredients for a minute.
3. Cover the tofu with this mixture and place in the fridge to marinate for 1 hour.
4. In a container, combine the lemon juice, stevia, olive oil, Dijon mustard, salt, and pepper.
5. Stir in the lettuce, carrot, and onion; set aside.
6. Heat oil, cook the tofu on both sides for 6 minutes in total.
7. Remove to a plate.
8. In the buns, add the tofu and top with the slaw. Close the buns and serve.

Nutrition:
Calories: 315 kcal   **Fat:** 10.4 g   **Fiber:** 15.1 g   **Carbohydrates:** 9.4 g   **Protein:** 8.4 g

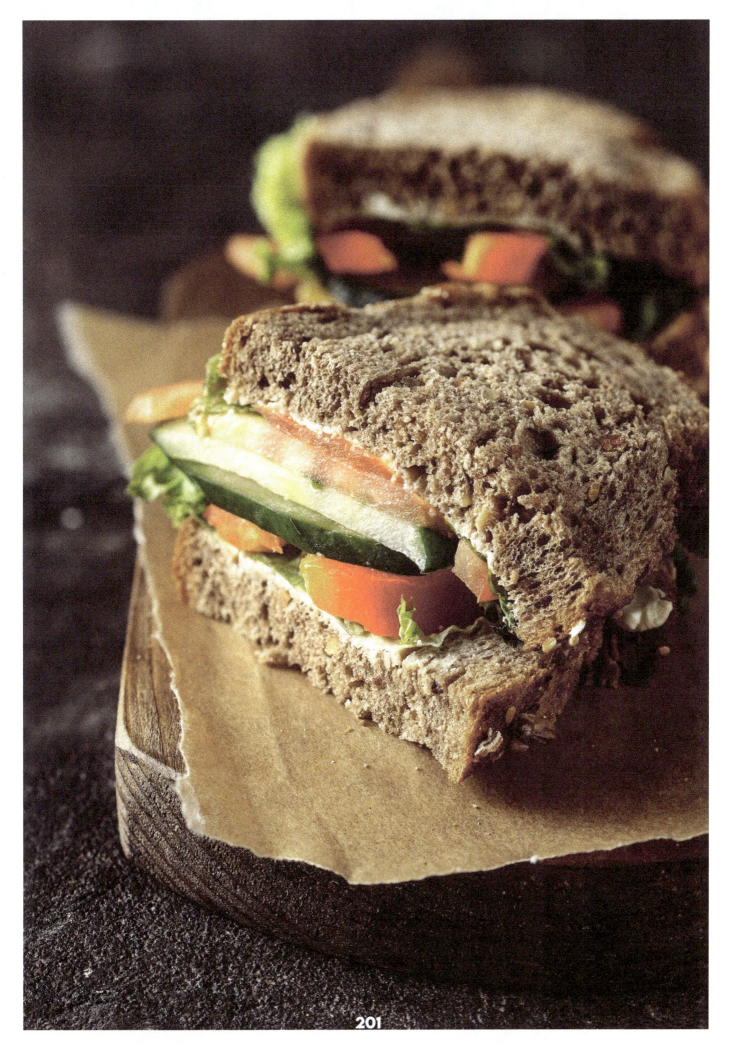

16

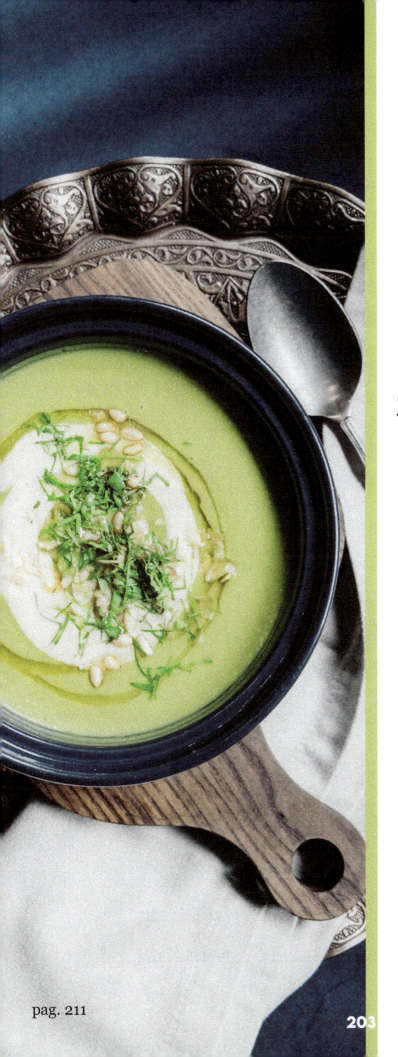

SOUP AND STEWS RECIPES

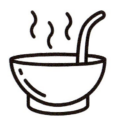

pag. 211

HEARTY FALL STEW

Prep Time: 15 min

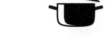
Cooking time: 8 hrs

Servings: 6

Ingredients:

- 3 tablespoons extra-virgin olive oil, divided
- 1 (2-pound / 907-g) beef chuck roast, cut into 1-inch chunks
- 1/2 teaspoon salt
- 1/4 teaspoon freshly ground black pepper
- 1/4 cup apple cider vinegar
- 1/2 sweet onion, chopped
- 1 cup diced tomatoes
- 1 teaspoon dried thyme
- 1 1/2 cups pumpkin, cut into 1-inch chunks
- 2 cups beef broth
- 2 teaspoons minced garlic
- 1 tablespoon chopped fresh parsley, for garnish

Directions:

1. Add the beef to the skillet, and sprinkle salt and pepper to season.
2. Cook the beef for 7 minutes or until well browned.
3. Put the cooked beef into the slow cooker and add the remaining ingredients, except for the parsley, to the slow cooker. Stir to mix well.
4. Slow cook for 8 hrs. and top with parsley before serving.

Nutrition:
Calories: 462 kcal **Fat:** 19.1 g **Fiber:** 11.6 g **Carbohydrates:** 10.7 g **Protein:** 18.6 g

COLD GREEN BEANS AND AVOCADO SOUP

Prep Time: 15 min   **Cooking time:** 15 min   **Servings:** 4

Ingredients:

- 1 tbsp. butter
- 2 tbsp. almond oil
- 1 garlic clove, minced
- 1 cup (227 g) green beans (fresh or frozen)
- 1/4 avocado
- 1 cup heavy cream
- 1/2 cup grated cheddar cheese + extra for garnish
- 1/2 tsp. coconut aminos
- Salt to taste

Directions:

1. Heat the butter and almond oil in a large skillet and sauté the garlic for 30 seconds.
2. Add the green beans and stir-fry for 10 minutes or until tender.
3. Add the mixture to a food processor and top with the avocado, heavy cream, cheddar cheese, coconut aminos, and salt.
4. Blend the ingredients until smooth.
5. Pour the soup into serving bowls, cover with plastic wraps and chill in the fridge for at least 2 hours.
6. Enjoy afterward with a garnish of grated white sharp cheddar cheese

Nutrition:
Calories: 301 kcal   **Fat:** 3.1 g   **Fiber:** 11.5 g   **Carbohydrates:** 2.8 g   **Protein:** 3.1 g

CHICKEN MUSHROOM SOUP

Prep Time: 15 min   **Cooking time:** 15 min   **Servings:** 4

Ingredients:

- 6 cups of chicken stock
- 5 slices of chopped bacon
- 4 cups cooked chicken breast, chopped
- 3 cups of water
- 2 cups of chopped celery root
- 2 cups of sliced yellow squash
- 2 tablespoons of olive oil
- 1/2 teaspoon of avocado oil
- 1/4 cup of chopped basil
- 1/4 cup of chopped onion
- 1/4 cup of chopped tomatoes
- 1 tablespoon of ground garlic
- 1 cup of sliced white mushrooms
- 1 cup green beans
- Salt
- Black pepper

Directions:

1. Heat oil in a skillet, add in half of the onions, sauté until soft.
2. Put in bacon and fry for a minute and a half.
3. Then, add in onions, garlic, tomatoes, and mushrooms, stir fry for three minutes.
4. Put in stock and fat water with the rest of the ingredients. Let it simmer for 10-15 minutes. Serve hot.

Nutrition:
Calories: 268 kcal   **Fat:** 10.5 g   **Fiber:** 4.9 g   **Carbohydrates:** 3.1 g   **Protein:** 12.9 g

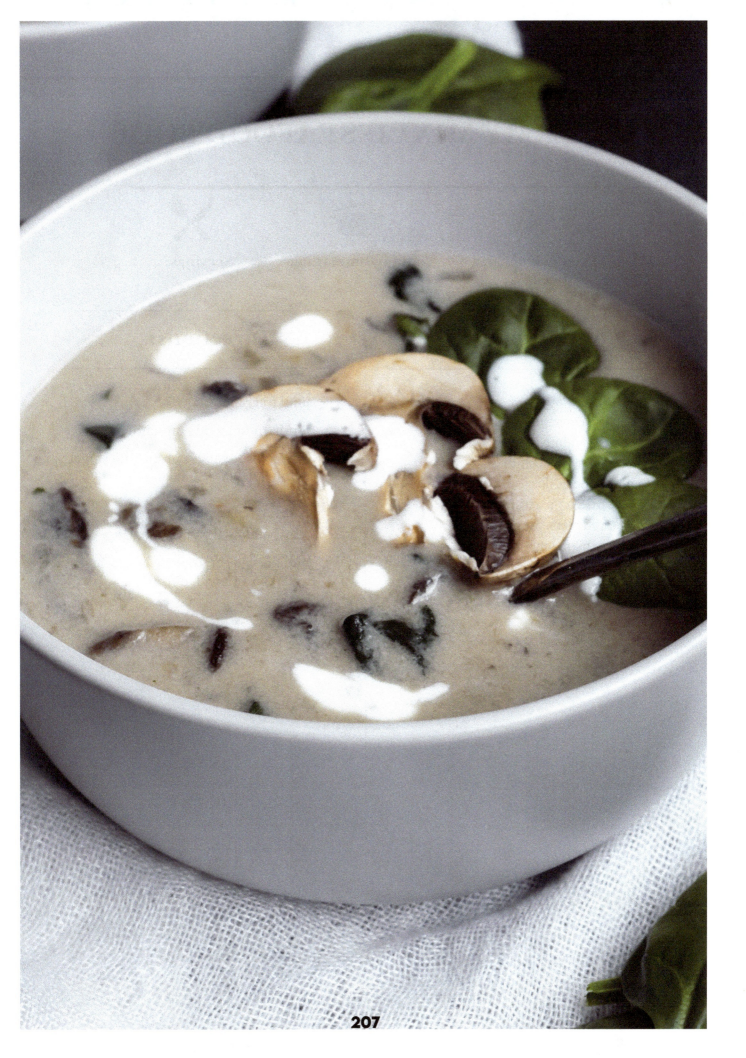

CREAMY MIXED SEAFOOD SOUP

Prep Time: 15 min **Cooking time:** 15 min **Servings:** 4

Ingredients:

- 1 tbsp. avocado oil
- 2 garlic cloves, minced
- 3/4 tbsp. almond flour
- 1 cup vegetable broth
- 1 tsp. dried dill
- 1 lb. frozen mixed seafood
- Salt and black pepper to taste
- 1 tbsp. plain vinegar
- 2 cups cooking cream
- Fresh dill leaves to garnish

Directions:

1. Heat oil sauté the garlic for 30 seconds or until fragrant.
2. Stir in the almond flour until brown.
3. Mix in the vegetable broth until smooth and stir in the dill, seafood mix, salt, and black pepper.
4. Bring the soup to a boil and then simmer for 3 to 4 minutes or until the seafood cooks.
5. Add the vinegar, cooking cream, and stir well. Garnish with dill, serve.

Nutrition:
Calories: 361 kcal **Fat:** 12.4 g **Fiber:** 8.5 g **Carbohydrates:** 3.9 g **Protein:** 11.7 g

ROASTED TOMATO AND CHEDDAR SOUP

Prep Time: 10 min   **Cooking time:** 15/20 min   **Servings:** 4

Ingredients:

- 2 tbsp. butter
- 2 medium yellow onions, sliced
- 4 garlic cloves, minced
- 5 thyme sprigs
- 8 basil leaves + extra for garnish
- 8 tomatoes
- 1/2 tsp. red chili flakes
- 2 cups vegetable broth
- Salt and black pepper to taste
- 1 cup grated cheddar cheese (white and sharp)

Directions:

1. Melt the butter in a pot and sauté the onions and garlic for 3 minutes or until softened.
2. Stir in the thyme, basil, tomatoes, red chili flakes, and vegetable broth.
3. Season with salt and black pepper.
4. Boil it then simmer for 10 minutes or until the tomatoes soften.
5. Puree all ingredients until smooth. Season.
6. Garnish with the cheddar cheese and basil. Serve warm.

Nutrition:
Calories: 341 kcal   **Fat:** 12.9 g   **Fiber:** 9.6 g   **Carbohydrates:** 4.8 g   **Protein:** 4.1 g

CAULIFLOWER KALE SOUP

 Prep Time: 10 min

 Cooking time: 50 min

 Servings: 4

Ingredients:

- 4 cups cauliflower florets
- 6 cups vegetable stock
- 1 tbsp. garlic, minced
- 1/4 cup onion, chopped
- 6 oz kale, chopped
- 6 tbsp. olive oil
- Pepper
- Salt

Directions:

1. Preheat the oven to 425 F.
2. Spread cauliflower onto the baking tray and drizzle with two tablespoons of oil and season with pepper and salt.
3. Roast cauliflower in a preheated oven for 25 minutes. Remove from the oven and set aside.
4. In a bowl, toss kale with two tablespoons of oil and season with salt. Arrange kale onto the baking tray and bake at 300 F for 30 minutes. Toss halfway through.
5. Heat oil.
6. Add onion and sauté for 3-4 minutes. Add garlic and sauté for a minute.
7. Add stock and roasted cauliflower and bring to boil.
8. Simmer it for 10 minutes.
9. Add kale and cook for 10 minutes more.
10. Puree the soup until smooth.
11. Serve and enjoy.

Nutrition:
Calories: 287 kcal **Fat:** 15.1 g **Fiber:** 4.1 g **Carbohydrates:** 3.1 g **Protein:** 5.8 g

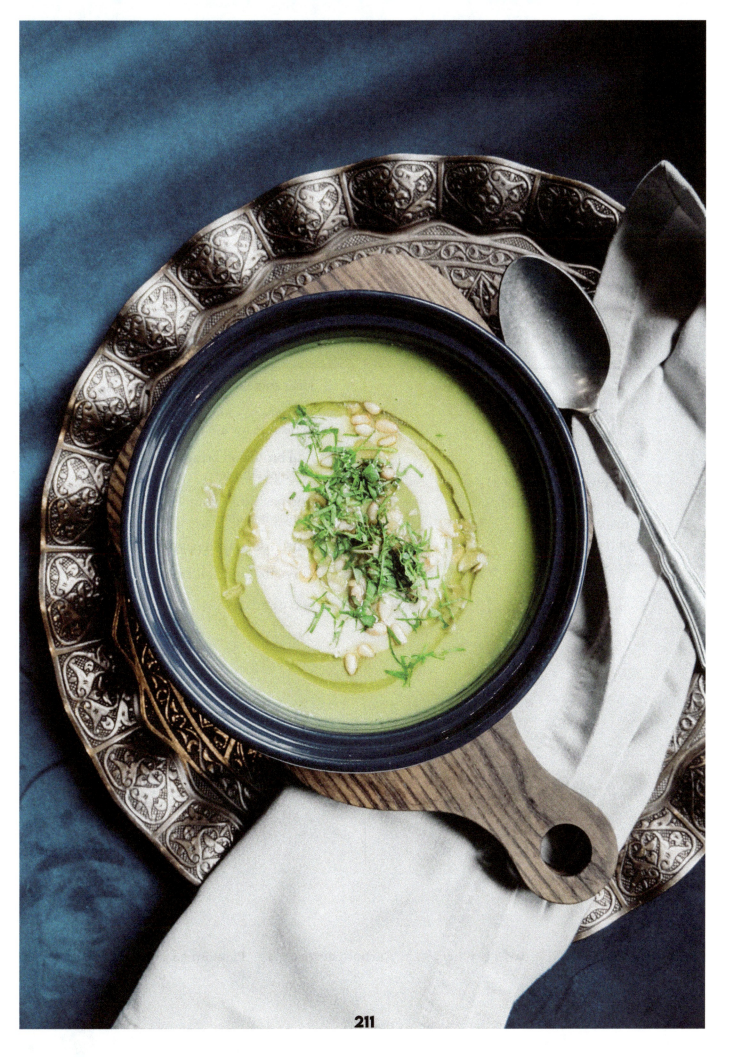

HEALTHY CELERY SOUP

Prep Time: 10 min   **Cooking time:** 20 min   **Servings:** 4

Ingredients:

- 3 cups celery, chopped
- 1 cup vegetable broth
- 5 oz cream cheese
- 1 1/2 tbsp. fresh basil, chopped
- 1/4 cup onion, chopped
- 1 tbsp. garlic, chopped
- 1 tbsp. olive oil
- 1/4 tsp. pepper
- 1/2 tsp. salt

Directions:

1. Heat some oil.
2. Add celery, onion and garlic to the saucepan and sauté for 4-5 minutes or until softened.
3. Add broth and bring to boil. Turn heat to low and simmer.
4. Add basil and cream cheese and stir until cheese is melted.
5. Season soup with pepper and salt.
6. Puree the soup until smooth.
7. Serve and enjoy.

Nutrition:
Calories: 201 kcal   **Fat:** 5.4 g   **Fiber:** 8.1 g   **Carbohydrates:** 3.9 g   **Protein:** 5.1 g

CREAMY ASPARAGUS SOUP

Prep Time: 10 min   **Cooking time:** 15 min   **Servings:** 4

Ingredients:

- 2 lbs. asparagus, cut the ends and chop into 1/2-inch pieces
- 2 tbsp. olive oil
- 3 garlic cloves, minced
- 2 oz parmesan cheese, grated
- 1/2 cup heavy cream
- 1/4 cup onion, chopped
- 4 cups vegetable stock
- Pepper
- Salt

Directions:

1. Heat olive oil in a large pot over medium heat.
2. Add onion to the pot and sauté until onion is softened.
3. Add asparagus and sauté for 2-3 minutes.
4. Add garlic and sauté for a minute. Season with pepper and salt.
5. Add stock and bring to boil. Turn heat to low and simmer until asparagus is tender.
6. Remove pot from heat and puree the soup using an immersion blender until creamy.
7. Return pot on heat. Add cream and stir well and cook over medium heat until just soup is hot. Do not boil the soup.
8. Remove from heat. Add cheese and stir well.
9. Serve and enjoy.

Nutrition:
Calories: 202 kcal   **Fat:** 8.4 g   **Fiber:** 6.1 g   **Carbohydrates:** 3.1 g   **Protein:** 5.3 g

COCONUT CURRY CAULIFLOWER SOUP

Prep Time: 15 min **Cooking time:** 30 min **Servings:** 4

Ingredients:

- 1 tbsp. olive oil
- 2-3 tsp. curry powder
- 1 medium onion
- 2 tsp. ground cumin
- 3 garlic cloves
- 1/2 tsp. turmeric powder
- 1 tsp. ginger
- 14 oz coconut milk
- 14 oz tomatoes
- 1 cup vegetable broth
- 1 cauliflower
- Salt and pepper

Directions:

1. Take a pot, adds olive oil and onion, and set it on a medium flame for sautéing.
2. After 3 minutes, add garlic, ginger, curry powder, cumin, and turmeric powder and sauté for more than 5 minutes.
3. Now add coconut milk, tomatoes, vegetable broth, and cauliflower and mix it well.
4. Let the mixture heat and bring to boil.
5. Now on low flame, cook it for at least 20 minutes until cauliflower turns into soft, blend the mixture well through a blender and heat the soup for more 5 minutes and add salt and pepper as per taste, serve the hot seasonal soup.

Nutrition:
Calories: 281 kcal **Fat:** 8.1 g **Fiber:** 3.8 g **Carbohydrates:** 3.2 g **Protein:** 4.8 g

GAZPACHO SOUP

Prep Time: 10 min   **Cooking time:** 15 min   **Servings:** 4

Ingredients:

- 1 large cucumber (to be sliced into chunks)
- 4 big ripe tomatoes (coarsely chopped)
- 1/2 bell pepper (any color)
- 2 cloves of garlic (minced)
- 1 celery rib (chopped)
- 1 tablespoon of lemon juice
- 1/4 tablespoon of celery pepper
- 1 tablespoon of fresh basil (chopped)
- 1 tablespoon of fresh parsley (chopped)
- Dash black pepper
- 1/2 tablespoon salt
- 3 tablespoons of red wine (vinegar/balsamic vinegar)
- 1/2 sweet onions (quartered)

Directions:

1. To make the gazpacho, place the cucumber chunks, chopped tomatoes, bell pepper, garlic, celery, lemon juice, and onion in the food processor or blender.
2. You may choose to blend or process in batches if needed
3. Add the vinegar (red/balsamic), salt, pepper to the blender or food processor and blend or process together until it is smooth or nearly smooth (the texture depends on you)
4. The next step is to pour soup into a serving bowl and stir in the fresh chopped parsley and basil
5. Cover the serving bowl with plastic wrap or foil or cover it with a plastic wrap and put the bowl inside the refrigerator for about 30 minutes or until when you are set to serve the gazpacho soup.
6. You can decide to add some extra fresh herbs to the soup for presentation as well as some avocado slices or crusty croutons
7. Serve gazpacho soup with a green salad, some artisanal or homemade bread as a substitute, balsamic vinegar, and olive oil for dipping for a light but a complete meal.
8. Serve and enjoy!

Nutrition:
Calories: 131 kcal   **Fat:** 9.4 g   **Fiber:** 16.8 g   **Carbohydrates:** 2.4 g   **Protein:** 4.1 g

NUTMEG PUMPKIN SOUP

Prep Time: 15 min   **Cooking time:** 20 min   **Servings:** 4

Ingredients:

- 1 tablespoon of butter
- 1 onion (diced)
- 1 16-ounce can of pumpkin puree
- 1 1/3 cups of vegetable broth
- 1/2 tablespoon of nutmeg
- 1/2 tablespoon of sugar
- Salt (to taste)
- Pepper (to taste)
- 3 cups of soymilk or any milk as a substitute

Directions:

1. Using a large saucepan, add onion to margarine and cook it between 3 and 5 minutes until the onion is clear
2. Add pumpkin puree, vegetable broth, sugar, pepper, and other ingredients and stir to combine.
3. Cook in medium heat for between 10 and fifteen minutes
4. Before serving the soup, taste and add more spices, pepper, and salt if necessary
5. Serve soup and enjoy it!

Nutrition:
Calories: 165 kcal   **Fat:** 4.9 g   **Fiber:** 11.9 g   **Carbohydrates:** 3.5 g   **Protein:** 4.2 g

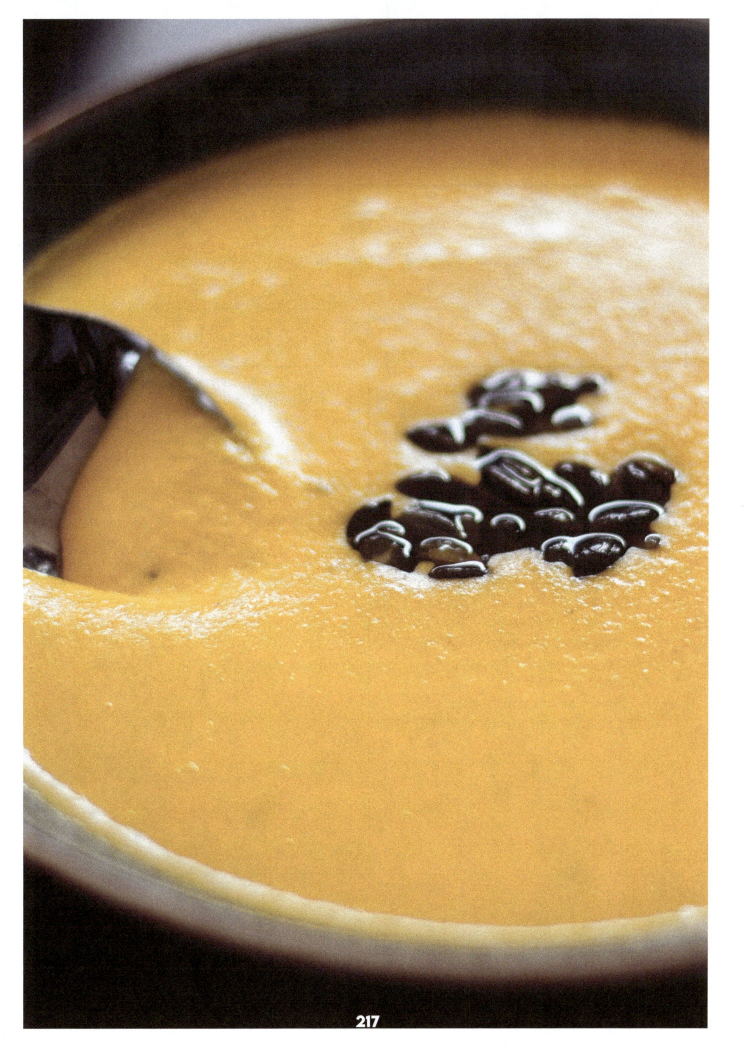

THAI COCONUT VEGETABLE SOUP

Prep Time: 15 min   **Cooking time:** 20 min   **Servings:** 4

Ingredients:

- 1 onion (diced)
- 2 bell peppers (red, diced)
- 1/4 teaspoon of cayenne
- 1/2 tablespoon of coriander
- 1/2 tablespoon of cumin
- 4 tablespoons of olive oil
- 1 can of chickpeas
- 1 carrot (sliced)
- 3 cloves of garlic
- 1/2 cup of basil or cilantro (fresh chopped)
- 1 teaspoon of salt
- 3 limes (freshly squeezed juice)
- 1/2 cup of vegetable broth
- 1 cup of coconut milk
- 1 cup of peanut butter
- 21/2 cups of tomatoes (finely diced)

Directions:

1. Sauté garlic and onions. Make ingredients to be soft for at least 3 to 5 minutes
2. Leaving out basil, add the rest of the ingredients and allow it to simmer. Cook over low heat for an hour
3. Put the half amount to the food processor, allow it to be very smooth, and return to the pot
4. Add either basil or cilantro, and your coconut food is ready. Before serving the soup, taste and add more seasoning if necessary. Serve, and enjoy!

Nutrition:
Calories: 151 kcal   **Fat:** 6.9 g   **Fiber:** 12.5 g   **Carbohydrates:** 3.1 g   **Protein:** 4.9 g

KETO CABBAGE SOUP

Prep Time: 10 min   **Cooking time:** 30 min   **Servings:** 6

Ingredients:

- 1/4 cup onion, diced
- 1 clove garlic, minced
- 1 tsp. cumin
- 1 head cabbage, chopped
- 1 1/4 cup canned diced tomatoes
- 5 oz. canned green chilis
- 4 cups vegetable stock
- Salt and pepper to taste

Directions:

1. Heat a heavy stockpot over medium-high heat. Add the onions and sauté for 5- 7 minutes more. Add the garlic and sauté for one more minute.

2. Bring this in to a low simmer and cook until the vegetables are tender about 30 minutes. And add water, if necessary, during cooking.

3. Transfer to serving bowls and serve hot.

Nutrition:
Calories: 131 kcal   **Fat:** 4.3 g   **Fiber:** 5.9 g   **Carbohydrates:** 1.2 g   **Protein:** 5.1 g

MIXED VEGETABLE STEW

 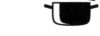

Prep Time: 15 min   **Cooking time:** 30 min   **Servings:** 6

Ingredients:

- 1 turnip, cut into bite-size pieces
- 1 onion, chopped
- 6 stalks celery, diced
- 1 carrot, sliced
- 15 oz. pumpkin puree
- 1 lb. green beans frozen or fresh
- 8 cups chicken stock
- 2 cups of water
- 1 Tbsp. fresh basil, chopped
- 1/4 tsp. thyme leaves
- 1/8 tsp. rubbed sage
- Salt to taste
- 1 lb. fresh spinach, chopped

Directions:

1. Put all the ingredients, excluding the spinach, into a heavy stockpot.
2. Bring to a low simmer and cook until the vegetables are tender about 30 minutes. Add water, if necessary, during cooking.
3. Add the spinach and stir until it's wilted about 5 minutes.
4. Transfer to serving bowls and serve hot.

Nutrition:
Calories: 198 kcal   **Fat:** 6.4 g   **Fiber:** 11.3 g   **Carbohydrates:** 2.5 g   **Protein:** 8.2 g

VEGETARIAN GREEN CHILI

Prep Time: 15 min   **Cooking time:** 20 min   **Servings:** 6

Ingredients:

- 3 tomatillos, sliced
- 3 jalapeno peppers, seeded and chopped
- 2 New Mexico green chili peppers, seeded and chopped
- 6 cloves garlic, minced
- 1 tomato, chopped
- 3 cups vegetable stock
- 2 tsp. cumin
- Salt and pepper to taste

Directions:

1. Put the tomatillos, jalapenos, New Mexico chilis, garlic, chicken stock, and tomato into a heavy stockpot.
2. Add the cumin, salt, and pepper on top of the meat.
3. Simmer and cook until fragrant, about 20 minutes. Add water, if necessary, during cooking.
4. Puree the soup until smooth.
5. Transfer the chili to serving bowls and serve hot,
6. garnished with chopped fresh cilantro.

Nutrition:
Calories: 201 kcal   **Fat:** 6.1 g   **Fiber:** 11.2 g   **Carbohydrates:** 2.1 g   **Protein:** 5.1 g

CHINESE TOFU SOUP

Prep Time: 5 min   **Cooking time:** 5 min   **Servings:** 2

Ingredients:

- 2 cups chicken stock
- 1 tbsp. soy sauce, sugar-free
- 2 spring onions, sliced
- 1 tsp. sesame oil, softened
- 2 eggs, beaten
- 1-inch piece ginger, grated
- Salt and black ground, to taste
- 1/2 pound extra-firm tofu, cubed
- A handful of fresh cilantros, chopped

Directions:

1. Boil in a pan over medium heat, soy sauce, chicken stock, and sesame oil.
2. Place in eggs as you whisk to incorporate thoroughly.
3. Change heat to low and add salt, spring onions, black pepper, ginger; cook for 5 minutes.
4. Place in tofu and simmer for 1 to 2 minutes.
5. Divide into soup bowls and serve sprinkled with fresh cilantro.

Nutrition:
Calories: 178 kcal   **Fat:** 4.1 g   **Fiber:** 3.1 g   **Carbohydrates:** 0.4 g   **Protein:** 5.5 g

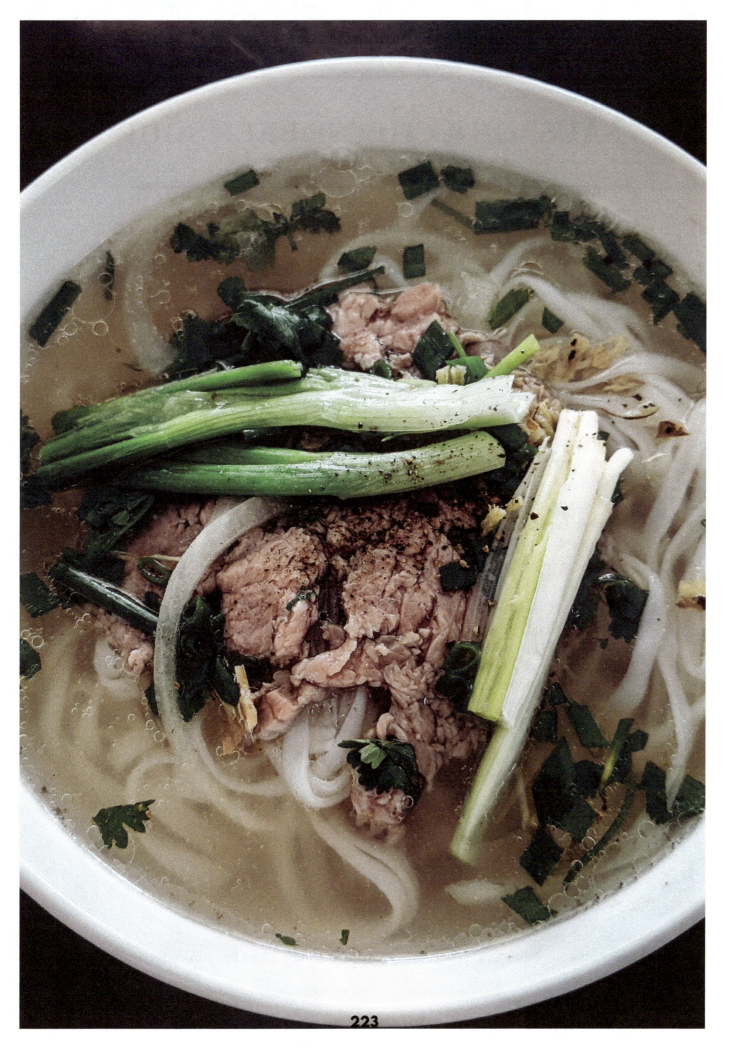

SAUSAGE & CHEESE BEER SOUP

 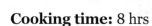

Prep Time: 15 min   **Cooking time:** 8 hrs   **Servings:** 4

Ingredients:

- 2 tbsp. butter
- 1/2 cup celery, chopped
- 1/2 cup heavy cream
- 5 oz turkey sausage, sliced
- 1 small carrot, chopped
- 2 garlic cloves, minced
- 4 ounces cream cheese
- 1/2 tsp. red pepper flakes
- 1 cup beer of choice
- 3 cups beef stock
- 1 yellow onion, diced
- 1 cup cheddar cheese, grated
- Kosher salt and black pepper, to taste
- Fresh parsley, chopped, to garnish

Directions:

1. To the crockpot, add butter, beef stock, beer, turkey sausage, carrot, onion, garlic, celery, salt, red pepper flakes, and black pepper, and stir to combine.
2. Cook for 6 hrs. on low.
3. Then add in the cream, cheddar, and cream cheese, and cook for two more hours.

Nutrition:
Calories: 345 kcal   **Fat:** 10.4 g   **Fiber:** 9.4 g   **Carbohydrates:** 4.1 g   **Protein:** 11.2 g

EGG DROP SOUP

Prep Time: 5 min   **Cooking time:** 10 min   **Servings:** 2

Ingredients:

- 4 cups chicken broth
- 1 teaspoon pink Himalayan sea salt
- 1/2 teaspoon ground ginger
- 1/2 teaspoon toasted sesame oil
- Pinch of ground white pepper
- 2 large eggs
- 1 scallion

Directions:

1. In a medium saucepan, combine the broth, salt, ginger, sesame oil, and white pepper.
2. Cook over medium-high heat until the soup is boiling.
3. In a small bowl, lightly beat the eggs.
4. Stirring the soup in a circular motion, slowly drizzle the beaten egg into the center of the vortex.
5. When all the egg is mixed in, stop stirring.
6. Cook for an additional 2 minutes, until the egg is cooked through, then pour into 2 bowls, sprinkle with the scallions, and serve.

Nutrition:
Calories: 121 kcal   **Fat:** 5.1 g   **Fiber:** 2.9 g   **Carbohydrates:** 1.2 g   **Protein:** 10 g

NEW ENGLAND CLAM CHOWDER

 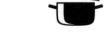

Prep Time: 15 min **Cooking time:** 25 min **Servings:** 2

Ingredients:

- 2 bacon slices, chopped
- 1 celery stalk, chopped
- 1/4 medium onion, chopped
- 1 garlic clove, minced
- 1 cup chicken broth
- 2 (6.5-ounce) cans chopped clams, drained, juices reserved
- 1 medium kohlrabi, peeled and cubed
- 1 bay leaf
- 1/2 teaspoon pink Himalayan sea salt
- 1/4 teaspoon freshly ground black pepper
- 1/4 teaspoon dried thyme
- Pinch of ground white pepper
- 1 1/2 cups decadent (whipping) cream

Directions:

1. Cook bacon
2. The pot with the bacon grease, sauté the celery and onion for 8 to 10 minutes until the onion is translucent. Add the garlic.
3. Add the broth, reserved clam juice (not the clams yet), the kohlrabi, bay leaf, salt, black pepper, thyme, and white pepper.
4. Simmer for 10 to 15 minutes, until the kohlrabi is tender.
5. Add the cream and clams. Stir to combine.
6. Simmer the soup for roughly 20 minutes, or until it reduces to your desired consistency.
7. Remove and discard the bay leaf.
8. Stir in the bacon crumbles and serve.

Nutrition:
Calories: 376 kcal **Fat:** 15.9 g **Fiber:** 10 g **Carbohydrates:** 4.1 g **Protein:** 13.1 g

CHICKEN NOODLE SOUP

Prep Time: 15 min   **Cooking time:** 25 min   **Servings:** 2

Ingredients:

- 1 tablespoon extra-virgin olive oil
- 8 ounces boneless, skinless chicken thighs, cubed
- 1/4 medium onion, chopped
- 1/2 celery stalk, thinly sliced
- 1 teaspoon minced garlic
- 2 cups chicken broth
- 1 teaspoon pink Himalayan sea salt
- 1/2 teaspoon freshly ground black pepper
- 1 teaspoon dried thyme
- 1 (7-ounce) package shirataki noodles, drained

Directions:

1. Heat oil.
2. Cook the chicken (10 minutes), until almost cooked through.
3. Put in celery, onion, and garlic. Cook for 7 to 10 minutes until the onion is translucent.
4. Pour the chicken broth into the pot. Add the salt, pepper, and thyme. Simmer for about 10 minutes.
5. Rinse the shirataki noodles, then add them to the pot right before serving.

Nutrition:
Calories: 368 kcal   **Fat:** 12.1 g   **Fiber:** 10.4 g   **Carbohydrates:** 3.1 g   **Protein:** 9.4 g

BROCCOLI CHEDDAR SOUP

 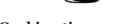

Prep Time: 15 min   **Cooking time:** 15 min   **Servings:** 2

Ingredients:

- 1/4 medium onion, chopped
- 2 tablespoons butter
- 1 garlic clove, minced
- 1 cup chicken broth
- 3/4 teaspoon pink Himalayan sea salt
- 1/2 teaspoon freshly ground black pepper
- 1/4 teaspoon dry mustard powder
- 8 ounces fresh broccoli florets, cooked and finely chopped
- 1 cup heavy (whipping) cream
- 1 cup shredded cheddar cheese

Directions:

1. In a medium pot, combine the onion, butter, and garlic over medium heat. Cook for 7 to 10 minutes until the onion is tender.
2. Add the broth, salt, pepper, and mustard, and bring the mixture to a boil.
3. Reduce the heat and add the broccoli and cream.
4. Slowly add the cheese, stirring. Serve.

Nutrition:
Calories: 317 kcal   **Fat:** 11.9 g   **Fiber:** 9.5 g   **Carbohydrates:** 4.3 g   **Protein:** 8.5 g

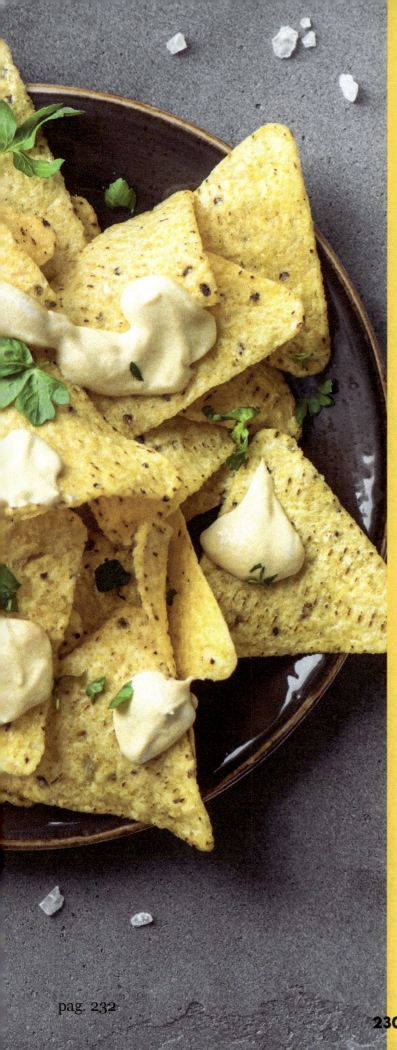

17

SNACKS RECIPES

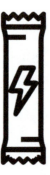

pag. 232

BLUEBERRY FAT BOMBS

Prep Time: 10 min   **Cooking time:** 0 min   **Servings:** 12

Ingredients:

- 1/2 cup blueberries, mashed
- 1/2 cup coconut oil, at room temperature
- 1/2 cup cream cheese, at room temperature
- 1 pinch nutmeg
- 6 drops liquid stevia

Directions:

1. Line the 12-cup muffin tin with 12 paper liners.
2. Put all the ingredients and process until it has a thick and mousse-like consistency.
3. Pour the mixture into the 12 cups of the muffin tin. Put the muffin tin into the refrigerate to chill for 1 to 3 hours.

Nutrition:
Calories: 120 kcal   **Fat:** 12.5 g   **Fiber:** 1.4 g   **Carbohydrates:** 2.1 g   **Protein:** 3.1 g

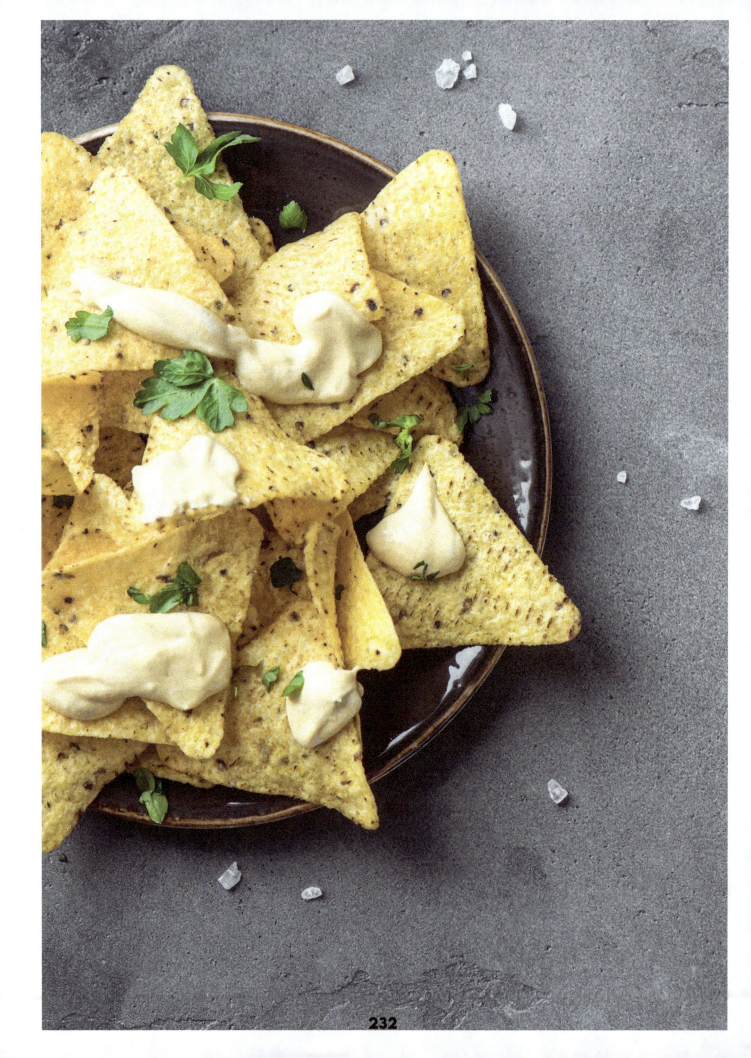

HERBED CHEESE CHIPS

Prep Time: 15 min   **Cooking time:** 15 min   **Servings:** 8

Ingredients:

- 3 tbsp. coconut flour
- 1/2 C. strong cheddar cheese, grated and divided
- 1/4 C. Parmesan cheese, grated
- 2 tbsp. butter, melted
- 1 organic egg
- 1 tsp. fresh thyme leaves, minced

Directions:

1. Preheat the oven to 350° F. Line a large baking sheet with parchment paper.
2. In a bowl, place the coconut flour, 1/4 C. of grated cheddar, Parmesan, butter, and egg and mix until well combined.
3. Make eight equal-sized balls from the mixture.
4. Arrange the balls onto a prepared baking sheet in a single layer about 2-inch apart.
5. Form into flat discs.
6. Sprinkle each disc with the remaining cheddar, followed by thyme.
7. Bake for around 15 minutes.

Nutrition:
Calories: 101 kcal   **Fat:** 6.5 g   **Fiber:** 1.4 g   **Carbohydrates:** 1.2 g   **Protein:** 3.1 g

CHEESY ZUCCHINI TRIANGLES WITH GARLIC MAYO DIP

Prep Time: 20 min   **Cooking time:** 30 min   **Servings:** 4

Ingredients:

- Garlic Mayo Dip:
- 1 cup crème Fraiche
- 1/3 cup mayonnaise
- 1/4 tsp. sugar-free maple syrup
- 1 garlic clove, pressed
- 1/2 tsp. vinegar
- Salt and black pepper to taste
- Cheesy Zucchini Triangles:
- 2 large zucchinis, grated
- 1 egg
- 1/4 cup almond flour
- 1/4 tsp. paprika powder
- 3/4 tsp. dried mixed herbs
- 1/4 tsp. swerve sugar
- 1/2 cup grated mozzarella cheese

Directions:

1. Start by making the dip; in a medium bowl, mix the crème Fraiche, mayonnaise, maple syrup, garlic, vinegar, salt, and black pepper.
2. Cover the bowl with a plastic wrap and refrigerate while you make the zucchinis.
3. Let the oven preheat at 400F. And line a baking tray with greaseproof paper. Set aside.
4. Put the zucchinis in a cheesecloth and press out as much liquid as possible.
5. Pour the zucchinis in a bowl.
6. Add the egg, almond flour, paprika, dried mixed herbs, and swerve sugar.
7. Mix well and spread the mixture on the baking tray into a round pizza-like piece with 1-inch thickness.
8. Let it bake for 25 minutes.
9. Reduce the oven's heat to 350°F/175°C, take out the tray, and sprinkle the zucchini with the mozzarella cheese.
10. Let it melt in the oven.
11. Remove afterward, set aside to cool for 5 minutes, and then slice the snacks into triangles.
12. Serve immediately with the garlic mayo dip.

Nutrition:
Calories: 286 kcal   **Fat:** 11.4 g   **Fiber:** 8.4 g   **Carbohydrates:** 4.3 g   **Protein:** 10.1 g

CRISPY PARMESAN CHIPS

 Prep Time: 10 min
 Cooking time: 5 min
 Servings: 8

Ingredients:

- 1 teaspoon butter
- 8 ounces full-fat Parmesan cheese, shredded or freshly grated

Directions:

1. Preheat the oven to 400°F.
2. The Parmesan cheese must be spooned onto the baking sheet in mounds, spread evenly apart.
3. Spread out the mounds with the back of a spoon until they are flat.
4. Bake the crackers until the edges are browned, and the centers are still pale about 5 minutes.

Nutrition:
Calories: 101 kcal   **Fat:** 9.4 g   **Fiber:** 3.1 g   **Carbohydrates:** 2.5 g   **Protein:** 1.2 g

KETO TRAIL MIX

Prep Time: 5 min   **Cooking time:** 0 min   **Servings:** 3

Ingredients:

- 1/2 cup salted pumpkin seeds
- 1/2 cup slivered almonds
- 3/4 cup roasted pecan halves
- 3/4 cup unsweetened cranberries
- 1 cup toasted coconut flakes

Directions:

1. In a skillet, place almonds and pecans. Heat for 2-3 minutes and let cool.
2. Once cooled, in a large resealable plastic bag, combine all ingredients.
3. Seal and shake vigorously to mix.
4. Evenly divide into suggested servings and store in airtight meal prep containers.

Nutrition:
Calories: 98 kcal **Fat:** 1.2 g **Fiber:** 4.1 g **Carbohydrates:** 1.1 g **Protein:** 3.2 g

TEX-MEX QUESO DIP

Prep Time: 5 min   **Cooking time:** 10 min   **Servings:** 6

Ingredients:

- 1/2 cup of coconut milk
- 1/2 jalapeño pepper, seeded and diced
- 1 teaspoon minced garlic
- 1/2 teaspoon onion powder
- 2 ounces goat cheese
- 6 ounces sharp Cheddar cheese, shredded
- 1/4 teaspoon cayenne pepper

Directions:

1. Preheat a pot then add the coconut milk, jalapeño, garlic, and onion powder.
2. Simmer then whisk in the goat cheese until smooth.
3. Add the Cheddar cheese and cayenne and whisk until the dip is thick, 30 seconds to 1 minute.

Nutrition:
Calories: 149 kcal   **Fat:** 12.1 g   **Fiber:** 3.1 g   **Carbohydrates:** 5.1 g   **Protein:** 4.2 g

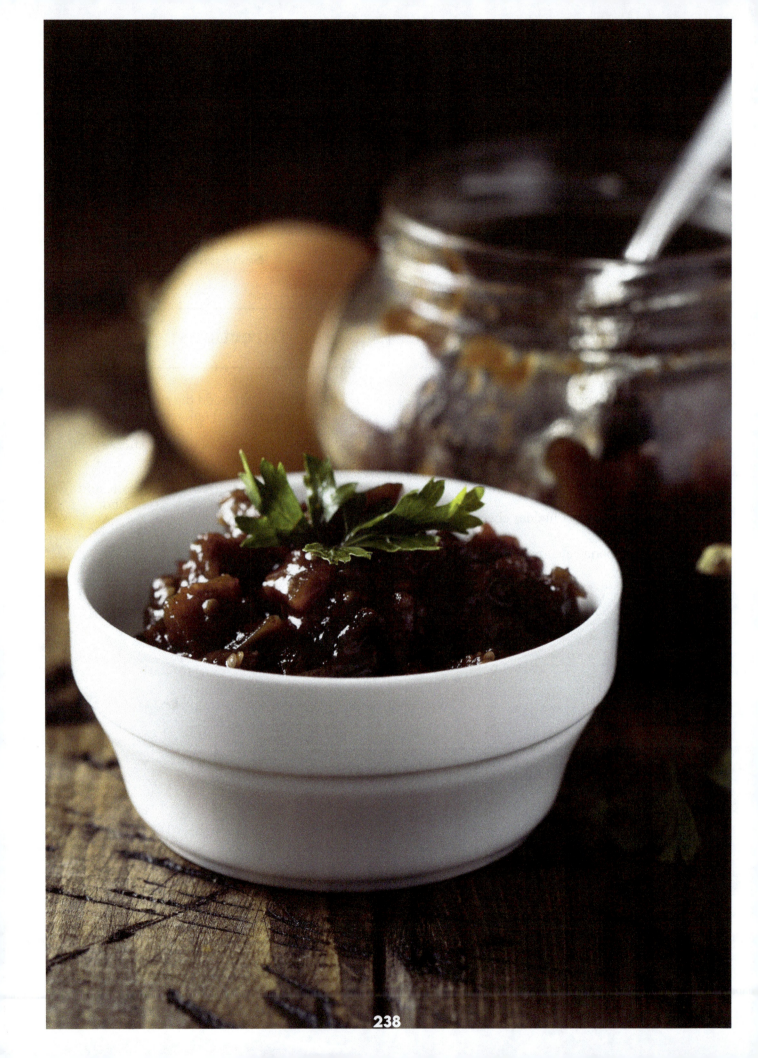

SWEET ONION DIP

Prep Time: 15 min   **Cooking time:** 25/30 min   **Servings:** 4

Ingredients:

- 3 cup sweet onion chopped
- 1 tsp. pepper sauce
- 2 cups Swiss cheese shredded
- Ground black pepper
- 2 cups mayonnaise
- 1/4 cup horseradish

Directions:

1. Take a bowl, add sweet onion, horseradish, pepper sauce, mayonnaise, and Swiss cheese, mix them well and transfer into the pie plate.
2. Preheat oven at 375.
3. Now put the plate into the oven and bake for 25 to 30 minutes until edges turn golden brown.
4. Sprinkle pepper to taste and serve with crackers.

Nutrition:
Calories: 278 kcal   **Fat:** 11.4 g   **Fiber:** 4.1 g   **Carbohydrates:** 2.9 g   **Protein:** 6.9 g

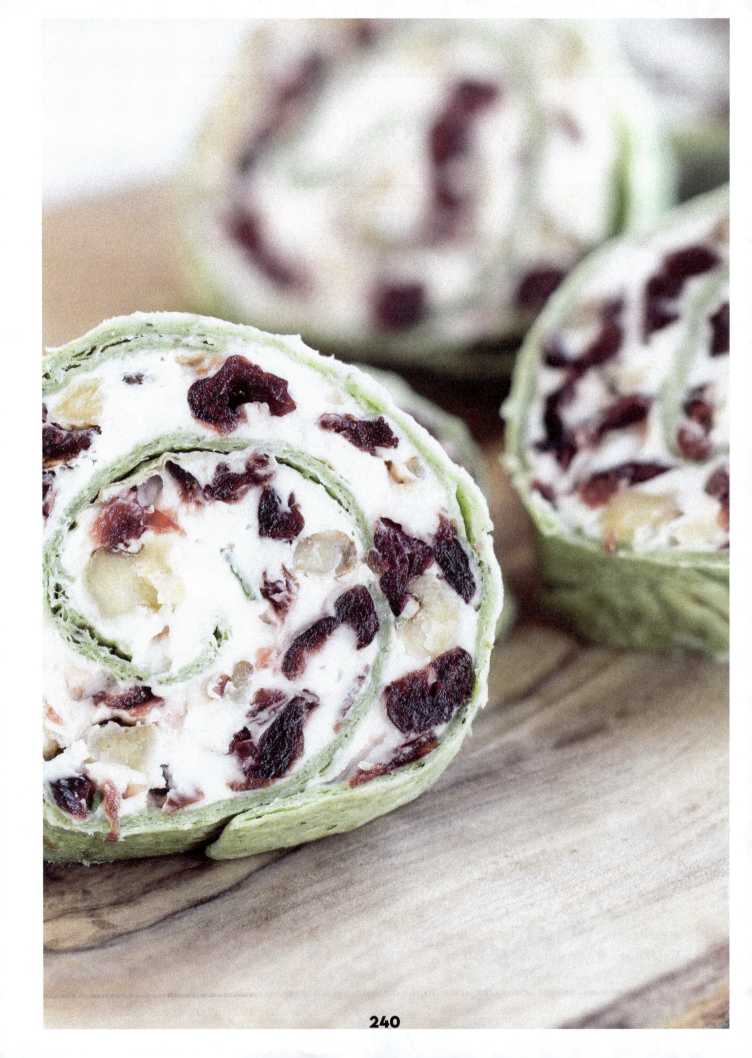

COLD CUTS AND CHEESE PINWHEELS

 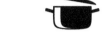

Prep Time: 20 min   **Cooking time:** 0 min   **Servings:** 2

Ingredients:

- 8 ounces cream cheese, at room temperature
- 1/4 pound salami, thinly sliced
- 2 tablespoons sliced pepperoncini

Directions:

1. Layout a sheet of plastic wrap on a large cutting board or counter.
2. Place the cream cheese in the center of the plastic wrap, and then add another layer of plastic wrap on top.
3. Using a rolling pin, roll the cream cheese until it is even and about 1/4 inch thick.
4. Try to make the shape somewhat resemble a rectangle.
5. Pull off the top layer of plastic wrap.
6. Place the salami slices so they overlap to cover the cream-cheese layer completely.
7. Place a new piece of plastic wrap on top of the salami layer to flip over your cream cheese–salami rectangle. Flip the layer, so the cream cheese side is up.
8. Remove the plastic wrap and add the sliced pepperoncini in a layer on top.
9. Roll the layered ingredients into a tight log, pressing the meat and cream cheese together. (You want it as tight as possible.)
10. Then wrap the roll with plastic wrap and refrigerate for at least 6 hours so it will set.
11. Slice and serve.

Nutrition:
Calories: 141 kcal   **Fat:** 4.9 g   **Fiber:** 2.1 g   **Carbohydrates:** 0.3 g   **Protein:** 8.5 g

KETO BREAD

Prep Time: 5 min **Cooking time:** 25 min **Servings:** 4

Ingredients:

- 5 tablespoons butter, at room temperature, divided
- 6 large eggs, lightly beaten
- 11/2 cups almond flour
- 3 teaspoons baking powder
- 1 tbsp. coconut oil
- Pinch pink Himalayan salt

Directions:

1. Preheat the oven to 390°F.
2. In a container, mix the eggs, almond flour, remaining four tablespoons of butter, baking powder, oil, and pink Himalayan salt until thoroughly blended. Pour into the prepared pan.
3. Bake for around 25 minutes.
4. Slice and serve.

Nutrition:
Calories: 121 kcal **Fat:** 4.3 g **Fiber:** 2.1 g **Carbohydrates:** 0.1 g **Protein:** 2.3 g

ZUCCHINI BALLS WITH CAPERS AND BACON

Prep Time: 3 hrs   **Cooking time:** 20 min   **Servings:** 10

Ingredients:

- 2 zucchinis, shredded
- 2 bacon slices, chopped
- 1/2 cup cream cheese, at room temperature
- 1 cup fontina cheese
- 1/4 cup capers
- 1 clove garlic, crushed
- 1/2 cup grated Parmesan cheese
- 1/2 tsp. poppy seeds
- 1/4 tsp. dried dill weed
- 1/2 tsp. onion powder
- Salt and black pepper, to taste
- 1 cup crushed pork rinds

Directions:

1. Preheat oven to 360 F.
2. Thoroughly mix zucchinis, capers, 1/2 of Parmesan cheese, garlic, cream cheese, bacon, and fontina cheese until well combined.
3. Shape the mixture into balls.
4. Refrigerate for 3 hours.
5. In a mixing bowl, mix the remaining Parmesan cheese, crushed pork rinds, dill, black pepper, onion powder, poppy seeds, and salt.
6. Roll cheese ball in Parmesan mixture to coat.
7. Arrange in a greased baking dish in a single layer and bake in the oven for 15-20 minutes, shaking once.

Nutrition:
Calories: 227 kcal   **Fat:** 12.5 g   **Fiber:** 9.4 g   **Carbohydrates:** 4.3 g   **Protein:** 14.5 g

STRAWBERRY FAT BOMBS

 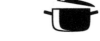

Prep Time: 30 min **Cooking time:** 0 min **Servings:** 6

Ingredients:

- 100 g strawberries
- 100 g cream cheese
- 50 g butter
- 2 tbsp. erythritol powder
- 1/2 teaspoon vanilla extract

Directions:

1. Put the cream cheese and butter (cut into small pieces) in a mixing bowl.
2. Let rest for 30 to 60 minutes at room temperature.
3. In the meantime, wash the strawberries and remove the green parts.
4. Pour into a bowl and process into a puree with a serving of oil or a mixer.
5. Add erythritol powder and vanilla extract and mix well.
6. Mix the strawberries with the other ingredients and make sure that they have reached room temperature.
7. Put the cream cheese and butter into a container.
8. Mix with a hand mixer or a food processor to a homogeneous mass.
9. Pour the mixture into small silicone muffin molds. Freeze.

Nutrition:
Calories: 95 kcal **Fat:** 9.1 g **Fiber:** 4.1 g **Carbohydrates:** 0.9 g **Protein:** 2.1 g

KALE CHIPS

Prep Time: 5 min   **Cooking time:** 25 min   **Servings:** 6

Ingredients:

- 400 g of kale
- 1 to 2 teaspoons of salt
- 2 tbsp. butter
- 50 g bacon fat

Directions:

1. Remove the stems and coarse ribs from the kale and tear the leaves into 5 cm pieces.
2. Wash the kale leaves thoroughly and dry them in a salad spinner.
3. Put the butter in a pan with the bacon fat and warm it up over low heat. Add salt and stir well.
4. Set aside and let cool.
5. Pack the kale in a zippered bag and pour the cooled, liquid mixture of bacon fat and butter into it.
6. Close the zippered bag and gently shake the kale leaves with the butter mixture. The leaves should take on a glossy color due to an even film of fat.
7. Place the kale leaves on a baking sheet and sprinkle with salt as desired.
8. Bake it for 25 minutes or until the leaves turn brown and crispy.
9. Let cool, divide into the recommended portions, and store in an airtight container.

Nutrition:
Calories: 59 kcal   **Fat:** 2.1 g   **Fiber:** 4.5 g   **Carbohydrates:** 0.9 g   **Protein:** 0.4 g

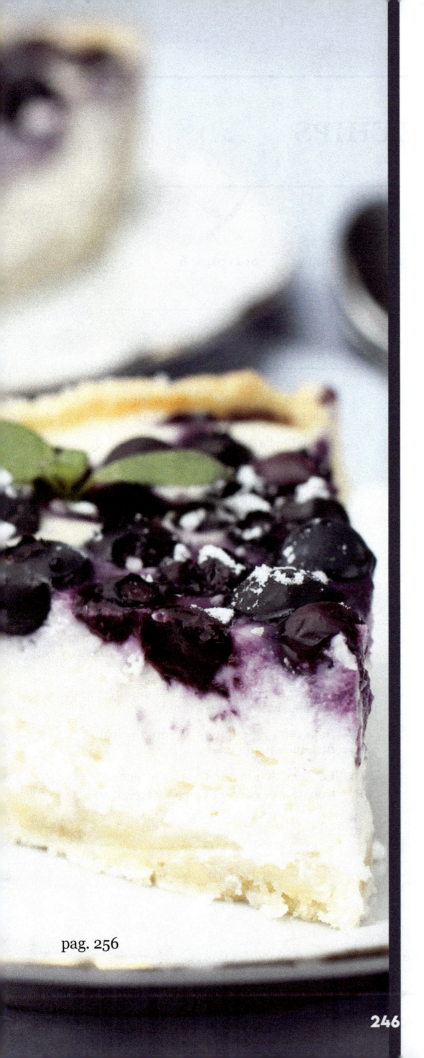

pag. 256

18

DESSERT RECIPES

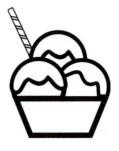

GREEN TEA AND MACADAMIA BROWNIES

Prep Time: 10 min   **Cooking time:** 20 min   **Servings:** 4

Ingredients:

- 4 tablespoons Swerve confectioners style sweetener
- 1/4 cup unsalted butter, melted
- Salt, to taste
- 1 egg
- 1 tablespoon tea matcha powder
- 1/4 cup coconut flour
- 1/2 teaspoon baking powder
- 1/2 cup chopped macadamia nuts

Directions:

1. Let the oven heat up to 350F.
2. Combine the sweetener, melted butter, and salt in a bowl. Stir to mix well.
3. Separate the egg into the bowl, whisk to combine well.
4. Fold in the matcha powder, coconut flour, and baking powder, then add the macadamia nuts. Stir to combine.
5. Pour the mixture on a baking sheet Level the mixture with a spoon to make sure it coats the bottom of the sheet evenly.
6. Bake for 18 minutes or until a sharp knife inserted in the center of the brownies comes out clean.
7. Remove the brownies from the oven and slice to serve.

Nutrition:
Calories: 241 kcal   **Fat:** 15.9 g   **Fiber:** 6 g   **Carbohydrates:** 12.1 g   **Protein:** 9.6 g

SESAME COOKIES

Prep Time: 15 min **Cooking time:** 15 min **Servings:** 12

Ingredients:

- 1/3 cup monk fruit sweetener, granulated
- 3/4 teaspoon baking powder
- 1 cup almond flour
- 1 egg
- 1 teaspoon toasted sesame oil
- 1/2 cup grass-fed butter, at room temperature
- 1/2 cup sesame seeds

Directions:

1. Let the oven heat up to 350F.
2. The dry ingredients must be combined in a bowl.
3. The wet ingredients must be mixed in a separate bowl.
4. Pour the wet mixture into the bowl for the dry ingredients. Stir until the mixture has a thick consistency and forms a dough.
5. Put the sesame seeds in a third bowl.
6. Divide and shape the dough into 16 1 1/2-inch balls, then dunk the balls in the bowl of sesame seeds to coat well.
7. Bash the balls until they are 1/2 inch thick, then put them on a baking sheet lined with parchment paper.
8. Keep a little space between each of them.
9. Baking Time (15 minutes)
10. Remove the cookies from the oven and allow to cool for a few minutes before serving.

Nutrition:
Calories: 174 kcal **Fat:** 12.4 g **Fiber:** 12.5 g **Carbohydrates:** 8.5 g **Protein:** 6.8 g

LEMON MUG CAKE

Prep Time: 5 min   **Cooking time:** 2 min   **Servings:** 1

Ingredients:

- 1 egg, lightly beaten
- 1/2 tsp. lemon rind
- 1 tbsp. butter, melted
- 1 1/2 tbsp. fresh lemon juice
- 2 tbsp. erythritol
- 1/4 tsp. baking powder, gluten-free
- 1/4 cup almond flour

Directions:

1. In a bowl or container, mix almond flour, baking powder, and sweetener.
2. Add egg, lemon juice, and melted butter in almond flour mixture and whisk until well combined.
3. Pour cake mixture into the microwave-safe mug and microwave for 90 seconds.
4. Serve and enjoy.

Nutrition:
Calories: 275 kcal   **Fat:** 5.9 g   **Fiber:** 2.4 g   **Carbohydrates:** 1.3 g   **Protein:** 4.1 g

ALMOND MILK PANNA COTTA

 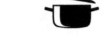

Prep Time: 15 min   **Cooking time:** 5 min   **Servings:** 4

Ingredients:

- 1 1/2 C. unsweetened almond milk, divided
- 1 tbsp. unflavored powdered gelatin
- 1 C. unsweetened coconut milk
- 1/3 C. Swerve
- 3 tbsp. cacao powder
- 2 tsp. instant coffee granules
- 6 drops liquid stevia

Directions:

1. In a large bowl, add 1/2 C. of almond milk and sprinkle evenly with gelatin.
2. Set aside until soaked.
3. In a pan, add the remaining almond milk, coconut milk, Swerve, cacao powder, coffee granules, and stevia and bring to a gentle boil, stirring continuously.
4. Remove from the heat.
5. In a blender, add the gelatin mixture and hot milk mixture and pulse until smooth.
6. Transfer the mixture into serving glasses and set aside to cool completely.
7. With plastic wrap, cover each glass and refrigerate for about 3-4 hours before serving.

Nutrition:
Calories: 190 kcal   **Fat:** 8.4 g   **Fiber:** 2.5 g   **Carbohydrates:** 1.5 g   **Protein:** 1.6 g

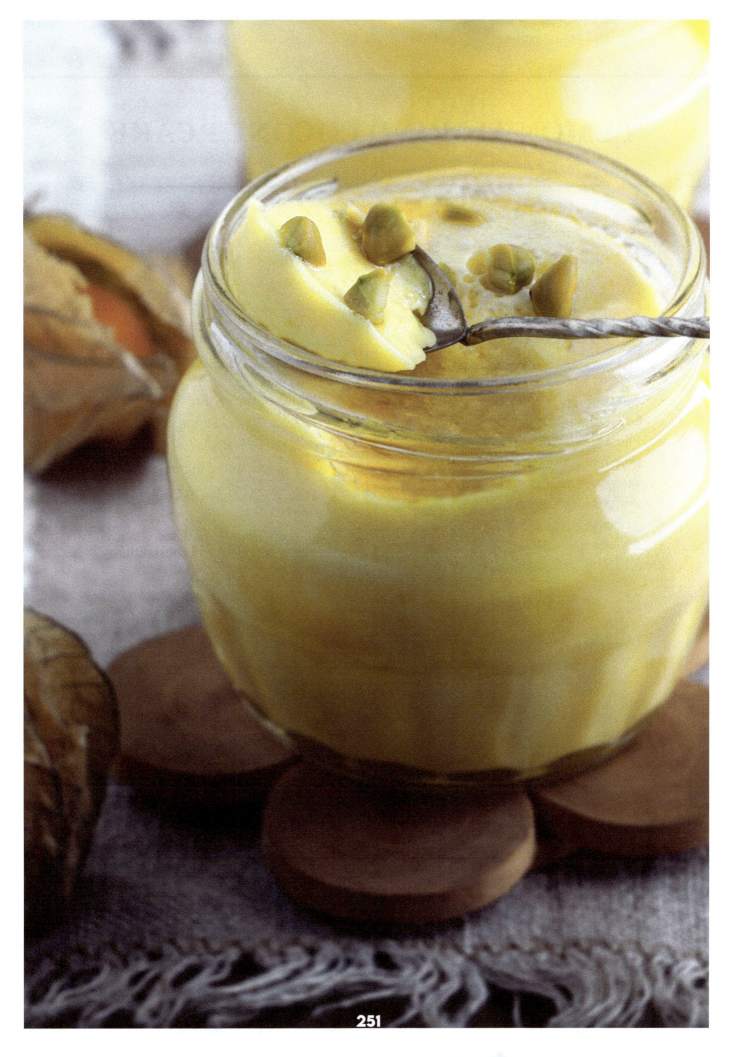

LEMON ALMOND COCONUT CAKE

Prep Time: 20 min   **Cooking time:** 40/45 min   **Servings:** 8

Ingredients:

- 250g almond
- 60g desiccated coconut
- Pinch of salt
- 150g natural sugar
- 1 teaspoon vanilla extract
- zest of 1 large lemon
- 3 eggs
- 200g butter, melted
- A handful of almond flakes

Directions:

1. Preheat oven to 180°C/360°F.
2. In a medium bowl, take almond, coconut, salt, sugar, vanilla, and lemon zest.
3. Mix in remaining ingredients.
4. Pour in a cake pan. Scatter with almond flakes.
5. Bake for approximately 40-45 minutes until lightly browned and cooked through the middle.

Nutrition:
Calories: 314 kcal   **Fat:** 12.4 g   **Fiber:** 6.1 g   **Carbohydrates:** 3.1 g   **Protein:** 3.9 g

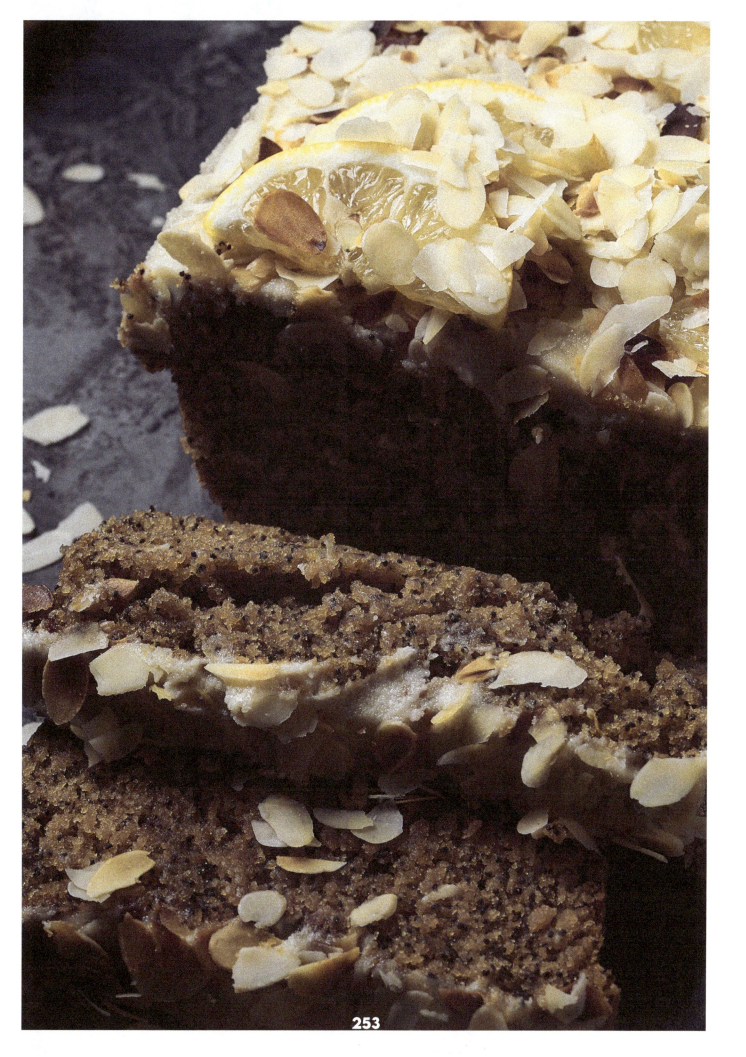

STRAWBERRY MOUSSE

Prep Time: 10 min **Cooking time:** 5 min **Servings:** 2

Ingredients:

- 1 cup heavy whipping cream
- 1 cup fresh strawberries, chopped
- 2 tbsp. Swerve
- 1 cup cream cheese

Directions:

1. Add heavy whipping cream in a bowl and beat until thickened using hand mixer.
2. Add sweetener and cream cheese and beat well.
3. Add strawberries and fold well.
4. Pour in serving glasses and place in the refrigerator for 1-2 hours.
5. Serve chilled and enjoy.

Nutrition:
Calories: 219 kcal **Fat:** 8 g **Fiber:** 3.1 g **Carbohydrates:** 1.9 g **Protein:** 1.2 g

PB& J CUPS

Prep Time: 20 min   **Cooking time:** 5 min   **Servings:** 4

Ingredients:

- 1/4 cup of water
- 1 teaspoon gelatin
- 3/4 cup of coconut oil
- 3/4 cup raspberries
- 6 to 8 tablespoon Stevia
- 3/4 cup peanut butter

Directions:

1. Line a muffin pan with parchment paper.
2. In a pan, combine the raspberries and water over medium heat.
3. Bring to a boil and then reduce the heat and let the water dry.
4. Mash the berries with a fork. Add in 2 to 4 tablespoons of the powdered sweetener.
5. Add in the gelatin and set aside to cool. Now make peanut butter mixture.
6. In the pan, put the peanut butter and coconut oil. Cook for 30 to 60 seconds, until melted.
7. Also, add in 2 to 4 tablespoons of the powdered sweetener.
8. Put half of the peanut butter mixture in a muffin pan and put in the freezer to firm up about 15 minutes.
9. Divide the raspberry mixture among the muffin cups and top with the remaining peanut butter mixture. Refrigerate until firm.

Nutrition:
Calories: 191 kcal **Fat:** 6.1 g **Fiber:** 2.2 g **Carbohydrates:** 1.8 g **Protein:** 3.1 g

MINI BLUEBERRY CHEESECAKES

 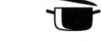

Prep Time: 35 min   **Cooking time:** 10 min   **Servings:** 6

Ingredients:

For crust:

- 1 cup almond flour
- 1 tbsp. sweetener
- 2 tbsp. coconut oil
- 1/4 tsp. vanilla extract
- Pinch of salt
- For cheesecake
- 8 oz cream cheese
- 1/2 cup sweetener
- 1 cup sour cream
- 1 tsp. vanilla extract
- Blueberry topping
- 1 cup fresh blueberries
- 2 tbsp. water
- 1/2 tbsp. lemon juice
- 1/4 tsp. xanthan gum

Directions:

1. For the crust: In a bowl, mix almond flour, sweetener, coconut oil, vanilla extract, and salt, stir well and make the dough.
2. Take muffin cups and place dough evenly in cups. Bake them for 8 minutes in a preheated oven at 325C until golden brown.
3. Cheesecake filling: in a bowl, have cream cheese and beat with an electric beater, now add sweetener and beat until turn fluffy.
4. In a bowl, mix sour cream and cheese cream mixture with vanilla extract and mix well.
5. Now fill the crust with cheesecake filling and cool for an hour.
6. Blueberry sauce: in a pan, put blueberries, water, and lemon juice and cook on medium flame, now turn flam low and add xanthan gum and stir for 2 to 3 minutes.

Nutrition:
Calories: 276 kcal   **Fat:** 10.4 g   **Fiber:** 2.3 g   **Carbohydrates:** 1.8 g   **Protein:** 3.8 g

CHOCOLATE WALNUT COOKIES

 Prep Time: 15 min   **Cooking time:** 12 min   **Servings:** 6

Ingredients:

- 1/4 cup coconut oil
- 3 tbsp. sweetener
- 4 tbsp. unsalted butter
- 1 cup sugar free chocolate chips
- 1 cup coconut flakes
- 1/2 cup pecans
- 1/2 cup walnuts
- 1 tsp. vanilla extract
- 4 egg yolks
- Sea salt

Directions:

1. Take a bowl and mix coconut oil, butter, sweetener, chocolate chips, vanilla extract, egg yolks, coconut, and walnuts and stir well.
2. Use a scope to make a cookie and drop an even amount of dough on the baking pan.
3. Sprinkle salt as per taste and bake for 12 minutes on preheated oven at 350F until golden brown.

Nutrition:
Calories: 231 kcal   **Fat:** 7.4 g   **Fiber:** 3.1 g   **Carbohydrates:** 2.8 g   **Protein:** 1.3 g

ALMOND SHORTBREAD COOKIES

Prep Time: 15 min   **Cooking time:** 12 min   **Servings:** 6

Ingredients:

For crust:

- 1/3 cup coconut flour
- 1/4 cup erythritol
- 2/3 cup almond flour
- 8 drops stevia
- 1/2 cup butter
- 1 tsp. almond or vanilla extract
- 1/4 tsp.. baking powder
- For glaze:
- 1/4 cup coconut butter
- 8 drops stevia

Directions:

1. In a bowl, add coconut flour, almond flour, erythritol, baking powder, and add vanilla or almond extract, stevia, and melted butter and make a soft dough.
2. The dough must be divided into two and chill in the refrigerator for 10 minutes.
3. Roll the dough on a sheet and cut cookies with the help of a cookie cutter.
4. Place cookies into a baking pan and bake for 6 minutes in a preheated oven at 180C.
5. Now let the cookies completely cool and apply the glaze.

Nutrition:
Calories: 245 kcal   **Fat:** 9.4 g   **Fiber:** 3.1 g   **Carbohydrates:** 2.9 g   **Protein:** 1.8 g

COCONUT CHIA PUDDING

Prep Time: 10 min   **Cooking time:** 0 min   **Servings:** 1

Ingredients:

- 1/4 cup chia seeds
- 1 1/4 cup coconut milk
- 2 tbsp. unsweetened coconut
- 1 tsp. vanilla extract
- 2 tbsp. maple syrup

Directions:

1. Soak chia seeds in water for 2 to 3 minutes.
2. Take a bowl, add coconut milk, maple syrup, vanilla extract, and chia seeds and whisk them well.
3. Let it aside and mix again after 5 minutes.
4. Put it in an airtight bag and place it in the refrigerator for 1 hour. Serve and enjoy chilled coconut chia pudding.

Nutrition:
Calories: 165 kcal   **Fat:** 1.4 g   **Fiber:** 5.4 g   **Carbohydrates:** 1.2 g   **Protein:** 3.1 g

BLACK BEAN BROWNIES

Prep Time: 15 min   **Cooking time:** 25 min   **Servings:** 12

Ingredients:

- 1 15-oz can of black beans
- 2 large flax eggs
- 3 tablespoon of coconut oil
- 3/4 cup cocoa powder
- 1/4 tablespoon of salt
- 1 tablespoon pure vanilla extract
- 1/2 cup of organic cane sugar
- 1 1/2 tablespoon of baking powder
- Toppings
- Crushed walnuts
- Pecans
- Daily-free semisweet chocolate chips

Directions:

1. Let the oven heat to 350F. prepare a baking dish lined with parchment paper.
2. Get a 12-slot standard size muffin pot and grease. Rinse your black beans well and drain.
3. Get the bowl of a food processor and prepare flax egg
4. Leave out walnuts and other toppings and add the remaining ingredients and puree
5. Get the muffin tin and pour the batter in it. Ensure that the top is smooth
6. Bake the batter until the tops are dry, and the edges start to pull away from the sides. This lasts 25 minutes.
7. Remove the pan and let it cool
8. Serve and enjoy!

Nutrition:
Calories: 259 kcal   **Fat:** 12.1 g   **Fiber:** 10.9 g   **Carbohydrates:** 3.8 g   **Protein:** 5.1 g

GRANNY SMITH APPLE TART

Prep Time: 15 min   **Cooking time:** 25 min   **Servings:** 6

Ingredients:

- 6 tbsp. butter
- 2 cups almond flour
- 1 tsp. cinnamon
- 1/3 cup sweetener
- Filling:
- 2 cups sliced Granny Smith
- 1/4 cup butter
- 1/4 cup sweetener
- 1/2 tsp. cinnamon
- 1/2 tsp. lemon juice
- Topping:
- 1/4 tsp. cinnamon
- 2 tbsp. sweetener

Directions:

1. Preheat oven to 370°F and combine all crust ingredients in a bowl.
2. Press this mixture into the bottom of a greased pan. Bake for 5 minutes.
3. Meanwhile, combine the apples and lemon juice in a bowl and sit until the crust is ready.
4. Arrange them on top of the crust.
5. Combine remaining filling ingredients, and brush this mixture over the apples. Bake for about 30 minutes.
6. Press the apples down with a spatula, return to oven, and bake for 20 more minutes. Combine the cinnamon and sweetener in a bowl, and sprinkle over the tart.

Nutrition:
Calories: 276 kcal   **Fat:** 11 g   **Fiber:** 10.4 g   **Carbohydrates:** 2.1 g   **Protein:** 3.1 g

COCONUT CHEESECAKE

Prep Time: 15 min   **Cooking time:** 25 min   **Servings:** 12

Ingredients:

- Crust:
- 2 egg whites
- 1/4 cup erythritol
- 3 cups desiccated coconut
- 1 tsp. coconut oil
- 1/4 cup melted butter
- Filling:
- 3 tbsp. lemon juice
- 6 ounces raspberries
- 2 cups erythritol
- 1 cup whipped cream
- Zest of 1 lemon
- 24 ounces cream cheese

Directions:

1. Line the pan with parchment paper. Preheat oven to 350°F and mix all crust ingredients.
2. Pour the crust into the pan. Bake for about 25 minutes; let cool.
3. Whisk the cream cheese in a container.
4. Add the lemon juice, zest, and erythritol. Fold in whipped cream mixture.
5. Fold in the raspberries gently. Spoon the filling into the crust.
6. Place in the fridge for 4 hours.

Nutrition:
Calories: 214 kcal   **Fat:** 11.4 g   **Fiber:** 8.4 g   **Carbohydrates:** 5.4 g   **Protein:** 9.1 g

CASHEW AND RASPBERRY TRUFFLES

Prep Time: 10 min

Cooking time: 0 min

Servings: 4

Ingredients:

- 2 cups raw cashews
- 2 tbsp. flax seed
- 1 1/2 cups sugar-free raspberry preserves
- 3 tbsp. swerve
- 10 oz unsweetened chocolate chips
- 3 tbsp. olive oil

Directions:

1. Grind the cashews and flax seeds in a blender for 45 seconds until smoothly crushed; add the raspberry and 2 tbsp. of swerve.
2. Process further for 1 minute until well combined. Form 1-inch balls of the mixture, place on the baking sheet, and freeze for 1 hour or until firmed up.
3. Melt the chocolate chips, oil, and 1tbsp. of swerve in a microwave for 1 1/2 minute.
4. Toss the truffles to coat in the chocolate mixture, put on the baking sheet, and freeze further for at least 2 hours

Nutrition:
Calories: 199 kcal   **Fat:** 4.1 g   **Fiber:** 3.1 g   **Carbohydrates:** 1 g   **Protein:** 3.2 g

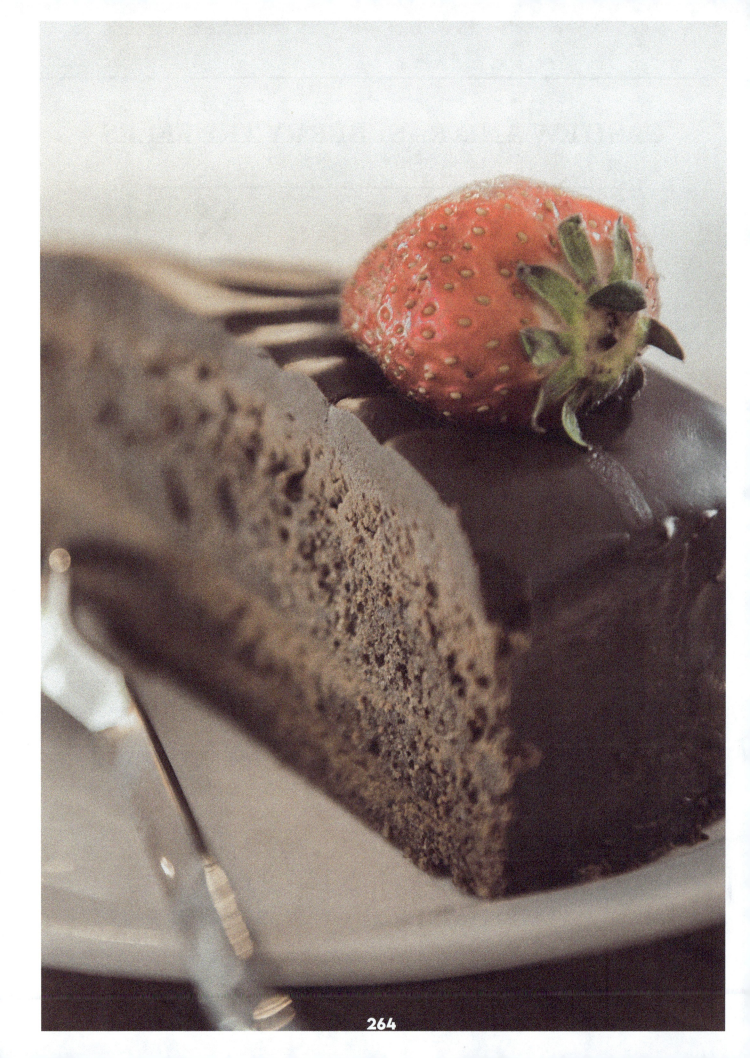

KETO CHOCOLATE CAKE

Prep Time: 20 min **Cooking time:** 17 min **Servings:** 4

Ingredients:

- 1/2 cup almond flour
- 1/4 cup xylitol
- 1 tsp. baking powder
- 1/2 tsp. baking soda
- 1 tsp. cinnamon, ground
- A pinch of salt
- A pinch of ground cloves
- 1/2 cup butter, melted
- 1/2 cup buttermilk
- 1 egg
- 1 tsp. pure almond extract
- For the Frosting:
- 1 cup heavy cream
- 1 cup dark chocolate, flaked

Directions:

1. Preheat oven to 360°F. Use a cooking spray to grease a donut pan.
2. In a bowl, mix the cloves, almond flour, baking powder, salt, baking soda, xylitol, and cinnamon.
3. In a separate bowl, combine the almond extract, butter, egg, and buttermilk.
4. Mix the wet mixture into the dry mixture. Evenly scoop the batter into the donut pan. Bake for 17 minutes.
5. Heat a pan and warm heavy cream; simmer for 2 minutes. Fold in the chocolate flakes; combine until all the chocolate melts; let cool. Put the frosting and serve.

Nutrition:
Calories: 289 kcal **Fat:** 15.1 g **Fiber:** 9.4 g **Carbohydrates:** 13.1 g **Protein:** 5.2 g

VANILLA FLAN

Prep Time: 15 min   **Cooking time:** 60 min   **Servings:** 4

Ingredients:

- 1/3 cup erythritol, for caramel
- 2 cups almond milk
- 4 eggs
- 1 tbsp. vanilla extract
- 1 tbsp. lemon zest
- 1/2 cup erythritol, for custard
- 2 cup heavy whipping cream
- Mint leaves, to serve

Directions:

1. Heat erythritol for the caramel in a deep pan. Add 2-3 tablespoons of water, and bring to a boil. Reduce the heat and cook until the caramel turns golden brown.
2. Divide between 4-6 metal tins. Set aside to cool.
3. In a bowl, mix eggs, remaining erythritol, lemon zest, and vanilla. Add almond milk and beat until well combined.
4. Pour the custard into each caramel-lined ramekin and place it in a deep baking tin.
5. Fill over the way with the remaining hot water. Bake at 345°F for 45-50 minutes.
6. Take out the ramekins and let cool for at least 4 hours in the fridge.
7. Run a knife slowly around the edges to invert onto a dish. Serve with dollops of whipped cream, scattered with mint leaves.

Nutrition:
Calories: 231 kcal   **Fat:** 10.3 g   **Fiber:** 4.1 g   **Carbohydrates:** 1.2 g   **Protein:** 3.7 g

BLUEBERRY CRISP

Prep Time: 15 min   **Cooking time:** 20 min   **Servings:** 2

Ingredients:

- 1/8 cup almond flour
- 1 cup fresh blueberries
- 2 tablespoons powdered swerve sweetener, divided
- 1/4 cup pecan halves
- 1 tablespoon ground flax
- 1/4 teaspoon salt
- 1/2 teaspoon ground cinnamon
- 1/2 teaspoon vanilla extract, unsweetened
- 2 tablespoons unsalted butter
- 2 tablespoons heavy cream, full-fat

Directions:

1. Preheat oven to 400°F.
2. Meanwhile, take two ramekins, fill each ramekin with 1/2 cup berries and 1/2 tablespoon sweetener, and stir until combined.
3. Place remaining ingredients into a food processor, pulse until combined, and then spoon this mixture evenly over berries.
4. Bake the berries for 15–20 minutes until the topping turns golden-brown and when done, top each with one tablespoon of heavy cream.
5. Serve straight away.

Nutrition:
Calories: 278 kcal   **Fat:** 11 g   **Fiber:** 6.4 g   **Carbohydrates:** 3.1 g   **Protein:** 6.2 g

LEMON COCONUT BALLS

Prep Time: 40 min   **Cooking time:** 0 min   **Servings:** 10

Ingredients:

- Balls
- 1/2 cup and 2 tablespoons almond flour
- 2 teaspoons Truvia
- 1/16 teaspoon salt
- 1 tablespoon Splenda sweetener
- 1/2 of a lemon, zested
- 1/4 cup cream cheese, full-fat, softened
- 2 teaspoons lemon juice
- 1/4 teaspoon vanilla extract, unsweetened
- 1 teaspoon sour cream, full-fat
- Coating
- 1 teaspoon Truvia
- 1/4 cup shredded coconut, unsweetened

Directions:

1. Prepare the balls and for this, take a medium-sized bowl, place all of its ingredients in it, and then stir well until the thick dough comes together.
2. Let the dough chill for 7 minutes.
3. Meanwhile, take a small bowl, place the coconut in it, add Truvia, and stir until mixed.
4. After 7 minutes, shape the dough into ten balls of even size and then roll them into coconut until well coated.
5. Arrange balls on a plate, freeze for a minimum of 30 minutes, and serve.

Nutrition:
Calories: 89 kcal   **Fat:** 6.1 g   **Fiber:** 4.2 g   **Carbohydrates:** 2.1 g   **Protein:** 4.1 g

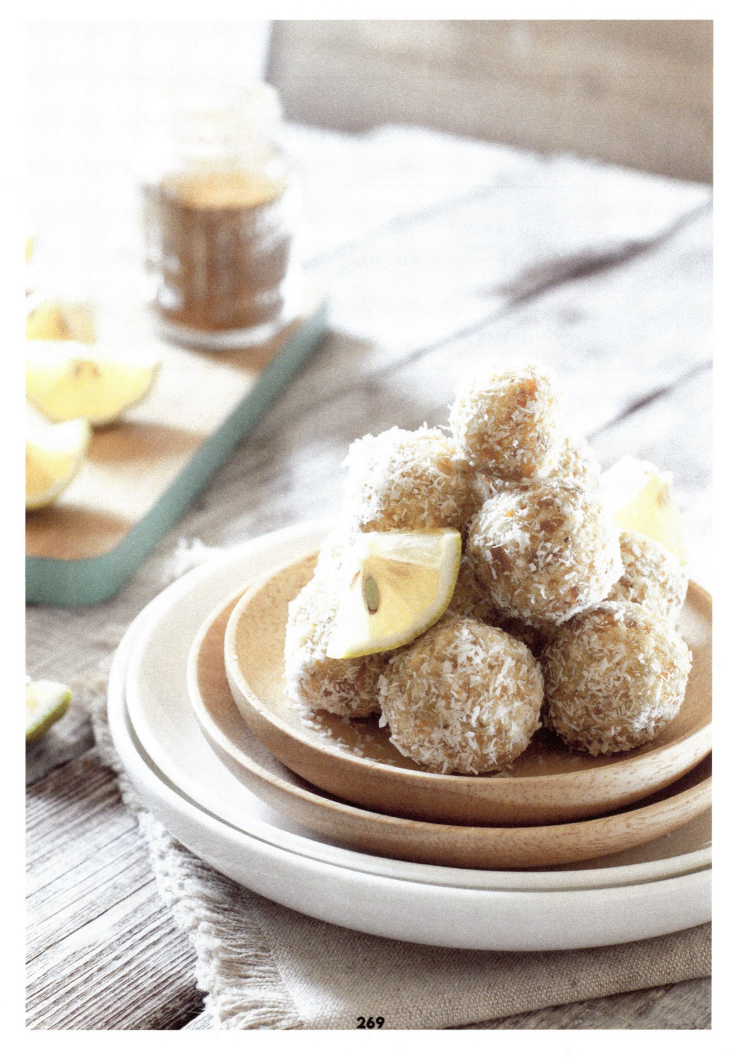

CHOCOLATE PUDDING

 Prep Time: 15 min

 Cooking time: 45 min

 Servings: 2

Ingredients:

- 1/2 teaspoon stevia powder
- 2 tablespoons cocoa powder
- 2 tablespoons water
- 1 tablespoon gelatin
- 1 cup of coconut milk
- 2 tablespoons maple syrup

Directions:

1. Heat pan with the coconut milk over medium heat; add stevia and cocoa powder and mix well.
2. In a bowl, mix gelatin with water; stir well and add to the pan.
3. Stir well, add maple syrup, whisk again, divide into ramekins and keep in the fridge for 45 minutes. Serve cold.

Nutrition:
Calories: 287 kcal **Fat:** 10.4 g **Fiber:** 9 g **Carbohydrates:** 2.1 g **Protein:** 3.1 g

SNICKERDOODLE MUFFINS

 Prep Time: 10 min

 Cooking time: 12 min

 Servings: 6

Ingredients:

- 6 2/3 tbsp. coconut flour
- 1/2 of egg
- 1 tbsp. butter, unsalted, melted
- 1 1/3 tbsp. whipping cream
- 1 tbsp. almond milk, unsweetened
- Others:
- 1 1/3 tbsp. erythritol sweetener and more for topping
- 1/4 tsp. baking powder
- 1/4 tsp. ground cinnamon and more for topping
- 1/4 tsp. vanilla extract, unsweetened

Directions:

1. Turn on the oven, and then set it to 350 degrees F and let it preheat.
2. Meanwhile, take a medium bowl, place flour in it, add cinnamon and baking powder. Stir until combined.
3. Take a separate bowl, place the half egg in it, add butter, sour cream, milk, and vanilla and whisk until blended.
4. Whisk in flour mixture until a smooth batter is obtained, divide the batter evenly between two silicon muffin cups and then sprinkle cinnamon and sweetener on top.
5. Bake the muffins for 10 to 12 minutes until firm, and then the top has turned golden brown and then serve and enjoy!

Nutrition:
Calories: 299 kcal **Fat:** 13.2 g **Fiber:** 10.5 g **Carbohydrates:** 4.1 g **Protein:** 3.8 g

CHOCOLATE AND STRAWBERRY CREPE

Prep Time: 10 min **Cooking time:** 12 min **Servings:** 4

Ingredients:

- 1 1/3 tbsp. coconut flour
- 1 tsp. of cocoa powder
- 1/4 tsp. flaxseed
- 1 egg
- 2 3/4 tbsp. coconut milk, unsweetened
- 2 tsp. avocado oil
- 1/8 tsp. baking powder
- 2 oz strawberry, sliced

Directions:

1. Take a medium bowl, place flour in it, and then stir in cocoa powder, baking powder, and flaxseed in it until mixed.
2. Add egg and milk and then whisk until smooth.
3. Take a medium skillet pan, place it over medium heat, add 1 tsp. oil and when hot, pour in half of the batter, spread it evenly, and then cook for 1 minute per side until firm.
4. Transfer crepe to a plate, add remaining oil, and cook another crepe using the remaining batter.
5. When done, fill crepes with strawberries, fold them and then serve and enjoy!

Nutrition:
Calories: 312 kcal **Fat:** 10.2 g **Fiber:** 5.4 g **Carbohydrates:** 3.1 g **Protein:** 5.2 g

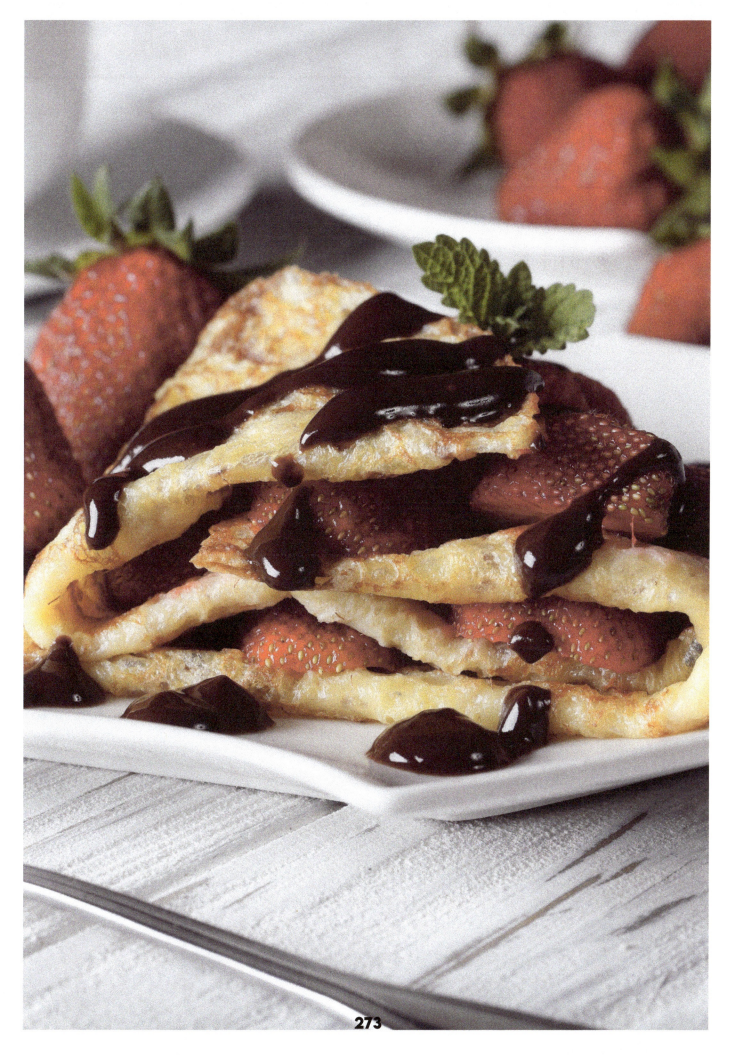

CREAM CHEESE AND PUMPKIN CUPS

Prep Time: 10 min   **Cooking time:** 12 min   **Servings:** 8

Ingredients:

- 4 tbsp. almond flour
- 1 1/3 tbsp. coconut flour
- 2 tbsp. pumpkin puree
- 2 2/3 tbsp. cream cheese, softened
- 1/2 of egg
- 2/3 tbsp. butter, unsalted
- 1/4 tsp. pumpkin spice
- 2/3 tsp. baking powder
- 2 tbsp. erythritol sweetener

Directions:

1. Turn on the oven, then set it to 350 degrees F and let it preheat.
2. Take a medium bowl, place butter and 1 1/2 tbsp. sweetener in it, and then beat until fluffy.
3. Take a medium bowl, place flours in it, stir in pumpkin spice, baking powder until mixed, mix all mixtures, then distribute it into two silicone muffin cups.
4. Take a medium bowl, place cream cheese in it, and stir in remaining sweetener until well combined.
5. Divide the cream cheese mixture into the silicone muffin cups, swirl the batter and cream cheese mixture using a toothpick and then bake for 10 to 12 minutes until muffins have turned firm.

Nutrition:
Calories: 289 kcal   **Fat:** 9.4 g   **Fiber:** 6.1 g   **Carbohydrates:** 3.1 g   **Protein:** 3.2 g

19

DRINKS

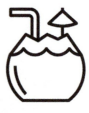

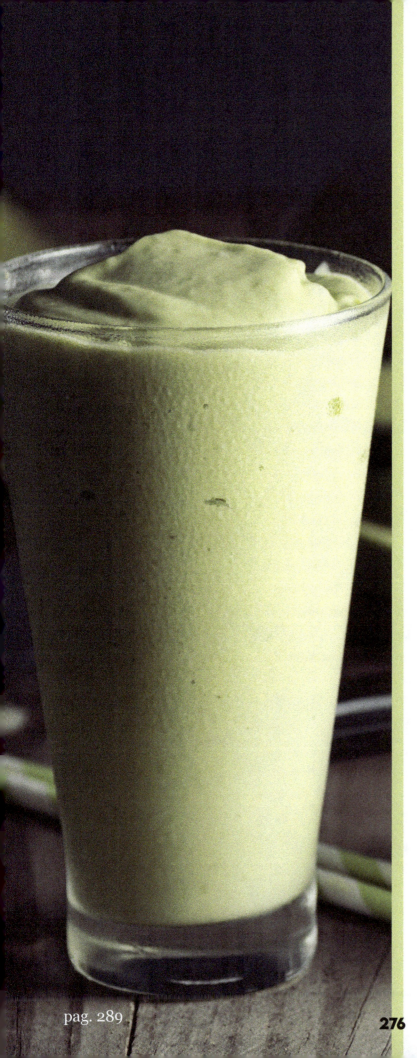

PUMPKIN SPICE LATTE

Prep Time: 5/10 min   **Cooking time:** 0 min   **Servings:** 1

Ingredients:

- 1 ounce of unsalted butter
- 2 tablespoons of pumpkin spice
- 2 tablespoons of instant coffee powder
- 1 cup of boiling water
- Heavy whipped cream

Directions:

1. Put all ingredients except cream inside a blender, and blend until the foam is formed.
2. Pour in a cup, and sprinkle cinnamon.
3. Add a dollop of cream and enjoy hot.

Nutrition:
Calories: 217 kcal   **Fat:** 12.9 g   **Fiber:** 2.3 g   **Carbohydrates:** 3.1 g   **Protein:** 4.1 g

BUTTER NUTMEG COFFEE

Prep Time: 5/10 min   **Cooking time:** 0 min   **Servings:** 1

Ingredients:

- 1 cup of coffee
- 2 tablespoons of ghee
- 1 tablespoon of coconut oil
- 1/2 teaspoon of nutmeg

Directions:

1. Pour coffee, ghee, oil, and nutmeg in a blender, and blend until smooth.
2. Serve hot.

Nutrition:
Calories: 210 kcal   **Fat:** 10 g   **Fiber:** 7.5 g   **Carbohydrates:** 3.1 g   **Protein:** 1.9 g

TROPICAL VANILLA MILKSHAKE

Prep Time: 15 min   **Cooking time:** 0 min   **Servings:** 1

Ingredients:

- 2 tablespoons of erythritol
- 1 cup of coconut milk
- 1/4 cup of heavy cream
- 1 teaspoon of vanilla extract

Directions:

1. Pour in the vanilla extract and erythritol into the blender.
2. Add in the coconut milk, then the heavy cream, and blend for 10 to 20 seconds.
3. Add ice if you'd like or freeze.

Nutrition:
Calories: 231 kcal   **Fat:** 9.5 g   **Fiber:** 3.1 g   **Carbohydrates:** 2.9 g   **Protein:** 4.2 g

CREAMY CINNAMON SMOOTHIE

 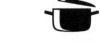

Prep Time: 15 min   **Cooking time:** 0 min   **Servings:** 2

Ingredients:

- 2 cups of coconut milk
- 1 scoop vanilla protein powder
- 5 drops liquid stevia
- 1 teaspoon ground cinnamon
- 1/2 teaspoon alcohol-free vanilla extract

Directions:

1. Put the coconut milk, protein powder, stevia, cinnamon, and vanilla in a blender and blend until smooth.
2. Pour into two glasses and serve immediately.

Nutrition:
Calories: 212 kcal   **Fat:** 3.1 g   **Fiber:** 5.2 g   **Carbohydrates:** 3.7 g   **Protein:** 4.1 g

BLUEBERRY TOFU SMOOTHIE

Prep Time: 15 min **Cooking time:** 0 min **Servings:** 1

Ingredients:

- 6 ounces of silken tofu
- 1 medium banana
- 2/3 cups of soy milk
- 1 cup of frozen or fresh blueberries (divided)
- 1 tablespoon of honey
- 2-3 ice cubes (optional)

Directions:

1. Drain the silken tofu to remove the excess water (silken tofu as a high-water content)
2. Peele and slice the banana. Place the sliced banana on a baking sheet and freeze them. This process usually takes up to 15 minutes. This helps to make the smoothie thicker.
3. Get a blender. Blend the banana, tofu, and soy milk. This usually takes up to 30 seconds.
4. Add 1/2 cup of the blueberries to the banana, tofu, and soymilk. Then blend it until it is very smooth.
5. Put the remaining blueberries. Add honey and ice cubes. Blend it until it is well combined.
6. Serve and enjoy.

Nutrition:
Calories: 312 kcal   **Fat:** 9.5 g   **Fiber:** 11.8 g   **Carbohydrates:** 2.7 g   **Protein:** 12.1 g

BULLETPROOF COFFEE

Prep Time: 5 min   **Cooking time:** 0 min   **Servings:** 1

Ingredients:

- 1 1/2 cups hot coffee
- 2 tablespoons MCT oil powder or Bulletproof Brain Octane Oil
- 2 tablespoons butter or ghee

Directions:

1. Pour the hot coffee into the blender.
2. Add the oil powder and butter, and blend until thoroughly mixed and frothy.
3. Pour into a large mug and enjoy.

Nutrition:
Calories: 245 kcal   **Fat:** 9.4 g   **Fiber:** 4.2 g   **Carbohydrates:** 1.2 g   **Protein:** 2.3 g

MORNING BERRY-GREEN SMOOTHIE

Prep Time: 15 min **Cooking time:** 0 min **Servings:** 4

Ingredients:

- 1 avocado, pitted and sliced
- 3 cups mixed blueberries and strawberries
- 2 cups unsweetened almond milk
- 6 tbsp. heavy cream
- 2 tsp. erythritol
- 1 cup of ice cubes
- 1/3 cup nuts and seeds mix

Directions:

1. Combine the avocado slices, blueberries, strawberries, almond milk, heavy cream, erythritol, ice cubes, nuts, and seeds in a smoothie maker; blend in high-speed until smooth and uniform.
2. Pour the smoothie into drinking glasses, and serve immediately.

Nutrition:
Calories: 290 kcal **Fat:** 5.1 g **Fiber:** 11 g **Carbohydrates:** 1.4 g **Protein:** 2 g

DARK CHOCOLATE SMOOTHIE

Prep Time: 10 min   **Cooking time:** 0 min   **Servings:** 2

Ingredients:

- 8 pecans
- 3/4 cup of coconut milk
- 1/4 cup of water
- 1 1/2 cups watercress
- 2 tsp. vegan protein powder
- 1 tbsp. chia seeds
- 1 tbsp. unsweetened cocoa powder
- 4 fresh dates, pitted

Directions:

1. In a blender, all ingredients must be blended until creamy and uniform. Place into two glasses and chill before serving.

Nutrition:
Calories: 299 kcal   **Fat:** 10 g   **Fiber:** 12.8 g   **Carbohydrates:** 2.1 g   **Protein:** 4.4 g

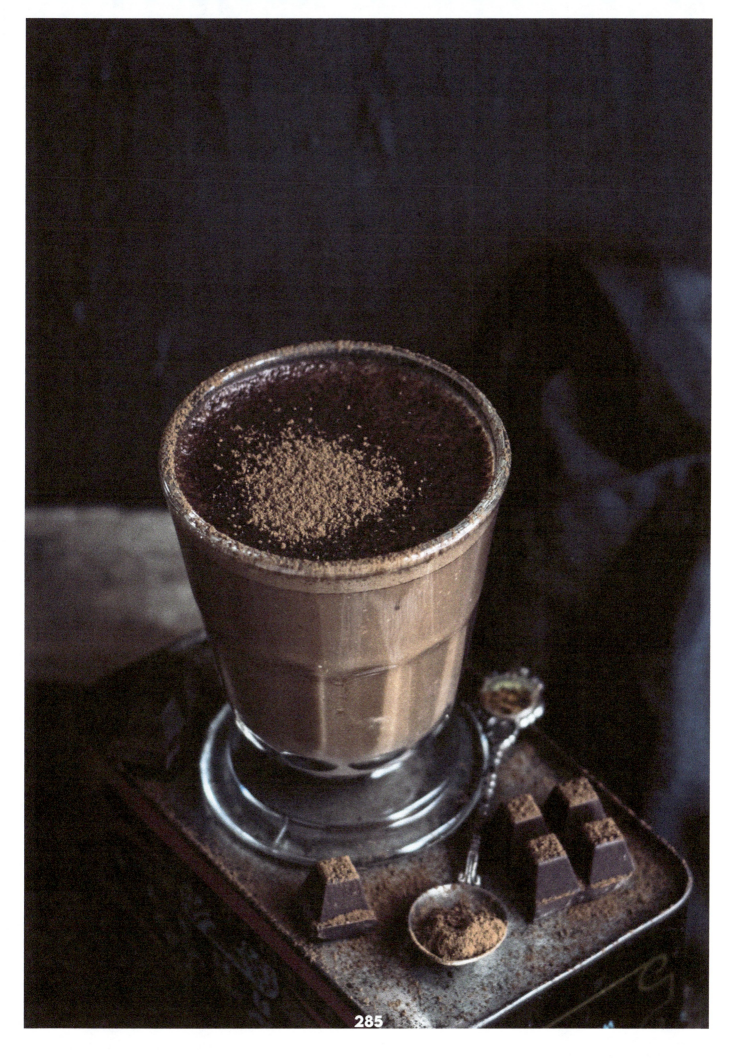

SUPER GREENS SMOOTHIE

Prep Time: 15 min   **Cooking time:** 0 min   **Servings:** 2

Ingredients:

- 6 kale leaves, chopped
- 3 stalks celery, chopped
- 1 ripe avocado, skinned, pitted, sliced
- 1 cup of ice cubes
- 2 cups spinach, chopped
- 1 large cucumber, peeled and chopped
- Chia seeds to garnish

Directions:

1. In a blender, add the kale, celery, avocado, and ice cubes, and blend for 45 seconds. Add the spinach and cucumber, and process for another 45 seconds until smooth.
2. Pour the smoothie into glasses, garnish with chia seeds, and serve the drink immediately

Nutrition:
Calories: 290 kcal   **Fat:** 9.4 g   **Fiber:** 12.1 g   **Carbohydrates:** 3.1 g   **Protein:** 8.5 g

KIWI COCONUT SMOOTHIE

 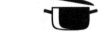

Prep Time: 5 min   **Cooking time:** 0 min   **Servings:** 2

Ingredients:

- 2 kiwis, pulp scooped
- 1 tbsp. xylitol
- 4 ice cubes
- 2 cups unsweetened coconut milk
- 1 cup of coconut yogurt
- Mint leaves to garnish

Directions:

1. Process the kiwis, xylitol, coconut milk, yogurt, and ice cubes in a blender, until smooth, for about 3 minutes.
2. Transfer to serving glasses, garnish with mint leaves, and serve.

Nutrition:
Calories: 298 kcal   **Fat:** 1.2 g   **Fiber:** 12.1 g   **Carbohydrates:** 1.2 g   **Protein:** 3.2 g

AVOCADO-COCONUT SHAKE

Prep Time: 5 min   **Cooking time:** 0 min   **Servings:** 2

Ingredients:

- 3 cups coconut milk, chilled
- 1 avocado, pitted, peeled, sliced
- 2 tbsp. erythritol
- Coconut cream for topping

Directions:

1. Combine coconut milk, avocado, and erythritol, into the smoothie maker, and blend for 1 minute to smooth. Pour the drink into serving glasses, add some coconut cream on top of them, and garnish with mint leaves. Serve immediately.

Nutrition:
Calories: 301 kcal   **Fat:** 6.4 g   **Fiber:** 12.9 g   **Carbohydrates:** 0.4 g   **Protein:** 3.1 g

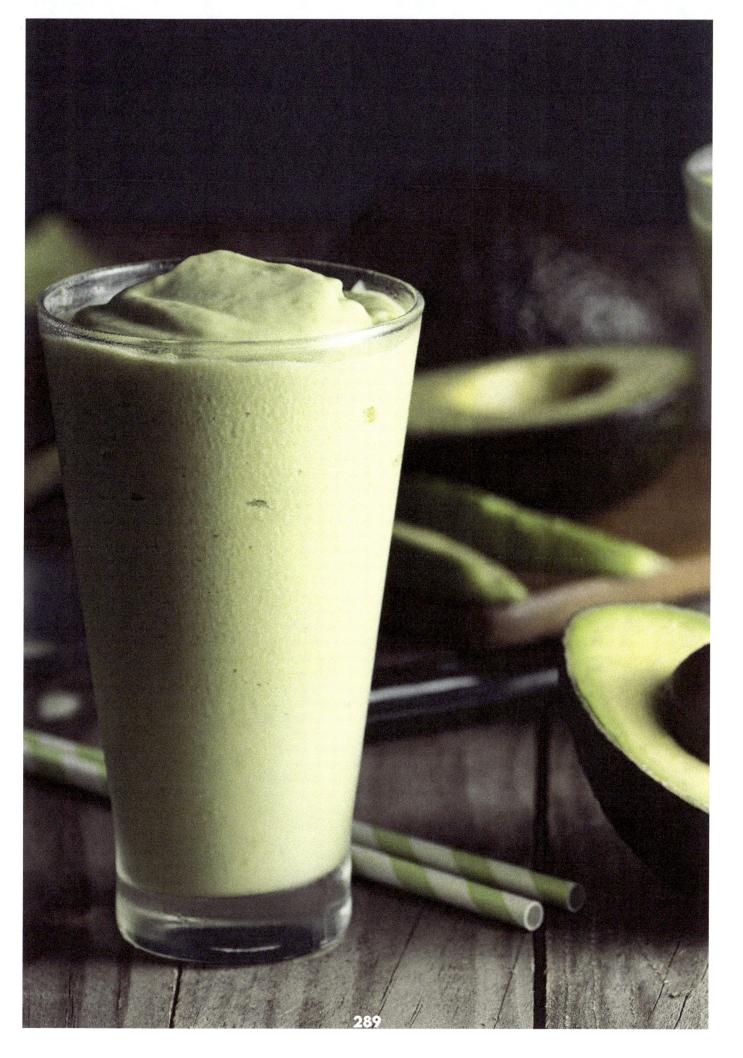

CREAMY VANILLA CAPPUCCINO

 Prep Time: 5 min

 Cooking time: 0 min

Servings: 2

Ingredients:

- 2 cups unsweetened vanilla almond milk, chilled
- 1 tsp. swerve sugar
- 1/2 tbsp. powdered coffee
- 1 cup cottage cheese, cold
- 1/2 tsp. vanilla bean paste
- 1/4 tsp. xanthan gum
- Unsweetened chocolate shavings to garnish

Directions:

1. In a blender, combine the almond milk, swerve sugar, cottage cheese, coffee, vanilla bean paste, and xanthan gum and process on high speed for 1 minute until smooth.

2. Pour into tall shake glasses, sprinkle with chocolate shavings, and serve immediately.

Nutrition:
Calories: 190 kcal **Fat:** 4.1 g **Fiber:** 1.1 g **Carbohydrates:** 0.5 g **Protein:** 2 g

GOLDEN TURMERIC LATTE WITH NUTMEG

Prep Time: 5 min   **Cooking time:** 5 min   **Servings:** 2

Ingredients:

- 2 cups almond milk
- 1/3 tsp. cinnamon powder
- 1/2 cup brewed coffee
- 1/4 tsp. turmeric powder
- 1 tsp. xylitol
- Nutmeg powder to garnish

Directions:

1. Add the almond milk, cinnamon powder, coffee, turmeric, and xylitol in the blender.
2. Blend the ingredients at medium speed for 50 seconds and pour the mixture into a saucepan.
3. Over low heat, set the pan and heat through for 6 minutes, without boiling.
4. Keep swirling the pan to prevent boiling. Turn the heat off, and serve in latte cups, topped with nutmeg powder.

Nutrition:
Calories: 254 kcal   **Fat:** 9.1 g   **Fiber:** 5 g   **Carbohydrates:** 1.2 g   **Protein:** 1 g

ALMOND SMOOTHIE

Prep Time: 5 min   **Cooking time:** 0 min   **Servings:** 2

Ingredients:

- 2 cups almond milk
- 2 tbsp. almond butter
- 1/2 cup Greek yogurt
- 1 tsp. almond extract
- 1 tsp. cinnamon
- 4 tbsp. flax meal
- 30 drops of stevia
- A handful of ice cubes

Directions:

1. Put the yogurt, almond milk, almond butter, flax meal, almond extract, collagen peptides, and stevia to the bowl of a blender.
2. Blend until uniform and smooth, for about 30 seconds.
3. Pour in smoothie glasses, add the ice cubes and sprinkle with cinnamon.

Nutrition:
Calories: 288 kcal   **Fat:** 6.4 g   **Fiber:** 11 g   **Carbohydrates:** 1 g   **Protein:** 1.4 g

RASPBERRY VANILLA SHAKE

Prep Time: 5 min   **Cooking time:** 0 min   **Servings:** 2

Ingredients:

- 2 cups raspberries
- 2 tbsp. erythritol
- 6 raspberries to garnish
- 1/2 cup cold unsweetened almond milk
- 2/3 tsp. vanilla extract
- 1/2 cup heavy whipping cream

Directions:

1. In a large blender, process the raspberries, milk, vanilla extract, whipping cream, and erythritol for 2 minutes; work in two batches if needed.
2. The shake should be frosty.
3. Pour into glasses, stick in straws, garnish with raspberries, and serve.

Nutrition:
Calories: 298 kcal   **Fat:** 5.1 g   **Fiber:** 11 g   **Carbohydrates:** 1.2 g   **Protein:** 1.4 g

BANANA SMOOTHIE

 Prep Time: 10 min   **Cooking time:** 0 min   **Servings:** 2

Ingredients:

- 1 1/2 cups unsweetened almond milk
- 1/2 cup heavy (whipping) cream
- 1 banana
- 2 scoops (25–28 grams) vanilla protein powder
- 2 tablespoons tahini
- 1/2 teaspoon ground cinnamon
- 5 ice cubes

Directions:

1. Blend the smoothie. Put the almond milk, cream, banana, protein powder, tahini, cinnamon, and ice in a blender and blend until smooth and creamy.
2. Serve. Pour into two tall glasses and serve.

Nutrition:
Calories: 308 kcal   **Fat:** 4.2 g   **Fiber:** 9.5 g   **Carbohydrates:** 2.2 g   **Protein:** 7.4 g

CREAMY MOCHA SMOOTHIE

Prep Time: 5 min   **Cooking time:** 0 min   **Servings:** 2

Ingredients:

- 2 cups strong-brewed coffee
- 1 cup unsweetened almond milk
- 1 cup unsweetened coconut milk
- 2 tablespoons chia seeds
- 2 tablespoons flaxseed meal
- 2 tablespoons coconut oil
- ⅛ teaspoon ground cinnamon
- Monk fruit sweetener, coarse, to taste

Directions:

1. Make coffee ice cubes. Pour the coffee into an ice tray and freeze for 4 hours minimum.
2. Blend the smoothie.
3. Put all of the coffee ice cubes (2 cups worth), almond milk, coconut milk, chia seeds, flaxseed meal, coconut oil, and cinnamon in a blender and blend smooth and creamy.
4. Add a sweetener. Serve.

Nutrition:
Calories: 315 kcal   **Fat:** 6.1 g   **Fiber:** 12 g   **Carbohydrates:** 1.2 g   **Protein:** 1.4 g

CONCLUSION

Thank you for making it through to the end of our book. Let's hope it was informative and able to provide you with all of the tools you need to achieve your goals in weight loss and a healthier lifestyle. Now that you are familiar with the Keto diet on many levels, you should feel confident in your ability to start your own Keto journey. This diet plan isn't going to hinder you or limit you, so do your best to keep this in mind as you begin changing your lifestyle and adjusting your eating habits. Packed with plenty of proteins and good fats, your body is going to go through a transformation as it works to see these things as energy. Before you know it, your body will have an automatically accessible reserve that you can utilize. Whether you need a boost of energy first thing in the morning or a second wind to keep you going throughout the day, this will already be inside of you.

As women grow older, there are a variety of changes occurring within their bodies. Having a great deal of impact, the reduction of estrogen often causes weight gain and a slower metabolism. The keto diet, with adjustments for the particular requirements of women over fifty years old, is a beautiful way to lose weight while relieving some of the aches and pains experienced as the lack of estrogen takes hold. By adapting the diet to make it more palatable for women over the age of 50, the ketogenic diet can be beneficial in more ways than just weight loss. Follow the principals of food choices suggested by studies performed around the world and reap the benefits of this popular diet. Ease into ketosis with the plan outlined, and you will find a smoother transition to a low-carbohydrate lifestyle. Use the tips and tricks to smooth over rough spots and use the food list to try new foods.

While on the Keto diet, you are building up energy stores for your body to utilize. This means that you should be feeling a necessary boost in your energy levels and the ability to get through each moment of each day without struggling. You can say goodbye to the sluggish feeling that often accompanies other diet plans. When you are on Keto, you should only be experiencing the benefits of additional energy and unlimited potential. Your diet isn't going to always feel like a diet. After some time, you will realize that you enjoy eating a Keto menu very much. Because your body will be switching the way it metabolizes, it will also be switching what it craves. Don't be surprised if you end up craving fats and proteins as you progress on the Keto diet — this is what your body will eventually want.

Keto diet helps control blood sugar and improve nutrition, which in turn not only improves insulin response and resistance but also protects against memory loss, which is often a part of aging.

You have the tools to reach success losing weight on the keto diet. In the end, the weight loss will be a very generous reward you will enjoy. Thank you once again!